A Connoisseur's Guide to Cannaphrodisiacs

Cannabis Climax

BIANCA LATIMER

Table of Contents

Introduction

As the pace of cannabis legalization continues to accelerate all over the world, a true renaissance of recreational and medical use is taking place at the very same time.

In the wake of Viagra's enormous popularity, the international market has been inundated by a blizzard of purported natural sex enhancers. Some of these products are nothing but hype, yet the growing cannasexual culture that reports enhanced libido, improved sexual function, and increased pleasure is hard to ignore. Natural agents of desire have long been said to include everything from maca and yohimbe to horny goat weed and ginseng, all promising to put more fire into your sex life. For the time being it is cannabis that is significantly boosting the sexual pleasure of people all over the world.

Ten states have now given clearance to the concept of recreational marijuana, while more than 30 have put medical marijuana laws on the books. The tally of states that allow the use of marijuana is poised to jump in a big way again this year, and many are saying that 2019 will be the biggest year yet in the grand scheme of cannabis reform. 95 percent of the U.S. population already lives in a state that grants some form of legal access to cannabis. Connecticut, Illinois, Minnesota, New Hampshire, New Jersey, New Mexico, New York, Rhode Island, Vermont are all likely to pass favourable new legislation this year, while the lawmakers of Kansas, Wisconsin, Texas, South Carolina are all said to favour decriminalisation. Looking ahead to 2020, states like Arizona, Florida, Ohio and North Dakota could consider ballot measures to fully legalize marijuana, while Mississippi, Nebraska and South Dakota might well see medical cannabis questions go before voters during that year's high-turnout presidential election. Already, some of the most likely contenders for the 2020 elections have lined up in support of legal cannabis, which has become a powerful campaign promise in recent years. As a result, some have already made up their minds: the next Democrat to get into office will make history by re-legalizing cannabis.

The South American nation of Uruguay was first to legalize cannabis in 2013. Across the pond, the Czech Republic, Spain, and Portugal have joined Holland in decriminalising personal use, while Germany has just legalized medical marijuana, a sign that other major European countries will be falling like dominoes soon. Colombia, Jamaica, Spain and Portugal are on the trajectory to become the next countries to legalize cannabis.

At first, I too had my doubts that cannabis could be an effective aphrodisiac but once I was introduced to its amazing powers, I became and immediate evangelist. Anything that can produce the longest and strongest orgasms I have ever experienced must have something to it. You might roll your eyes at the on-line reviews using words like "euphoria" and "life-changer" but until you try it for yourself, you will never know for sure.

That is why I have put this book together for you, so that you too can partake in the same mind-blowing tantric pleasure that the rest of us have already discovered. And if you are already a convert, then I hope that you will find plenty of new inspiration within these pages.

The Sexual Benefits of Cannabis

Most people agree that sex is extremely enjoyable. Most people that have tried, also agree that cannabis is equally enjoyable. It therefore makes perfect sense that combining the two together is going to bring about something quite special.

When asked if they have ever tried sex and cannabis at the same time, the vast majority usually reply in one of two ways. The first is "No, I have never tried that." The second is "Oh my God, I have such intensely awesome sex when I'm high!" The most significant thing here is that you will rarely, if ever hear a third reply of "Sex and cannabis, no way that was such a disaster."

Cannabis is a very efficient vasodilator, meaning that it enhances blood flow, which can be seen for example, in the way that your eyes go all blood-shot when you are stoned. This in turn increases engorgement, which is one of the things that naturally happens when your body physiologically responds to genital stimulation. Dilated capillaries in your erogenous zones means more blood flow and more oxygen to the area, which increases sensation. More blood flow means enhanced arousal and greater lubrication, and this is particularly effective on the vulva, which in reality, is in effect one big, exposed mucous membrane.

For both men and women, cannabis enhances the sensation of sex, making everything feel much more intense and hyper stimulated. Orgasms are more intense and even last longer than they do typically, with much higher peaks than are usually experienced.

Many women who feel sexually inhibited under normal conditions, but easily become sexually aroused when they are under the influence of cannabis. In practical terms, it helps you eliminate the things that are getting in the way of getting turned on. Things like stress, pain, anxiety, being stuck in your head and not feeling pleasurable sensations as readily in your body. Cannabis can help out with all of these problems. It relaxes you and contrary to popular belief actually reduces paranoia. This increased relaxation is one of the main reasons why women using cannabis are able to regularly achieve multiple orgasms. Some women even report that this is the only condition in which they manage to reach orgasm. Relaxed sex is good sex. ADD can also be a factor in some people's ability to just let go. They are just too distracted by everything else happening during sex to "focus," and even mistakenly brand themselves as being anorgasmic, when it is just a matter slowing down. A nice relaxing strain is the perfect way to achieve this.

Users of both sexes report that on many occasions erotic feelings are created for people they previously considered only as "friends." Alcohol also makes people more uninhibited, but its soporific qualities actually reduce blood flow making arousal harder to maintain, and even decreases any ability to climax. There is also a much greater instance of post-coital regret with drunken romps, as the booze not only reduces inhibition but it also affects selectivity. This often means that you often end up in boozy, one-night stands with random strangers, which is rarely successful.

Alcohol is currently the drug most widely used prior to sex. Many people lose their virginity drunk and quite a few pair booze and sex throughout their lives. Depending on one's weight and tolerance, two or more drinks increasingly depress the central nervous system. This raises the risk of erection impairment in men and reduced clitoral sensitivity in women. In both genders, drunk sex reduces the pleasure of orgasm and decreases sexual satisfaction. In addition, the combination of sex and alcohol greatly increases women's risk of sexual assault. So far, there is no evidence showing cannabis by itself being used as a date rape drug, despite fear-mongering anti-marijuana campaigns in Florida that try to prove otherwise.

Generally speaking, cannabis is sex-enhancing, while drunk sex is often lousy sex. Unlike alcohol, no study has ever shown cannabis to impair sexual function, nor has it been shown to increase risk of sexual assault. Users are still able to make good decisions on cannabis and maintain self-control, more so than when intoxicated on alcohol. Additionally, cannabis does not adversely affect memory of the interaction compared to alcohol. This leads to a lot more post-sex satisfaction than alcohol, so no more waking up and wondering who the hell that is lying next to you, and wondering what you spent all night doing with them. Unlike alcohol, which can take the wind out of my sexy sails, cannabis in the right dose actually does the opposite — it strengthens it. Also, unlike drunken sex, where there are sometimes gaps in my memory and lapses in my judgement; a cannabis high is measurable and sexy and never feels out of control. Of course, it is still a mind-altering substance, but you can remain present and aware. You will not lose yourselves, and that is what makes it so enjoyable. Best of all, it makes you feel amazing and, yet, you never get a hangover like you do with booze.

Cannabis not only increases pleasure it creates a greater appreciation of sexual activity as a means of communication, much stronger than any words or other actions. Participation in sexual activity involving cannabis can be particularly intimate and revealing, promoting trust and loving relationships.

Solo sexplorers on the other hand, often find that masturbating while tipsy can take forever and simply is not as enjoyable. Masturbating with the aid of cannabis feels fantastic. This is hardly a surprise as alcohol tends to numb sensation, while cannabis is well-known to enhance sensation. Cannabis allows individuals to become more present and aware of their bodies, especially with lower doses.

So what does bringing all that endo-cannabinoid positivity into the boudoir actually accomplish? Well, a good sativa is all about awakening, and sparkling creativity not like some debilitating West Coast skunk that makes you want to veg out of the couch and binge-watch Breaking Bad for hours on end. It has a uniquely energising effect, enabling marathon tantric sex sessions without the need for years of formal training and Yogic meditation. Cannaphrodisiacs are truly the female Viagra that we have all been waiting for. They offer an infinitely potent plant-based pleasure of the flesh, that is usually only seen in porno fantasy. Prepare yourself for multiple orgasms, hugely extended climaxes, and even squirting sessions for those who are physically capable. Both the quantity and quality of orgasms is vastly increased for male and female participants, but even more important are those previously rare life-changing experiences that alter the whole fabric of human consciousness. On one side of the Himalayan plateau, this is referred to as Samadhi, a oneness with the universe which comes with ultimate sexual pleasure.

For those of us living our boring rat-race lives in the heart of capitalist consumerism, this may all sound a little overblown, but

I can assure you that the human body is capable of far greater physical pleasure than most people believe is ever possible. Our current moral climate influenced by either protestant puritanism or fundamentalist Islamic dogma, simply does not allow for the possibility of an existence where life is one long extended act of sexual gratification. In fact, cultures where these kinds of exuberant lifestyles did exist have been largely expunged from our collective consciousness. One only needs to look at the amazing temple carvings of Khajurao in India to see that sex was at one time, exalted among all other human practices, or recall the free love societies of Polynesia which so captivated Fletcher Christian and his fellow mutineers, only to be erased from history by over-zealous missionaries and Calvinist despots.

The truth is that cannabis and sex are a classic combination. Both are gifts of nature, and we enjoy them because biology and evolution have designed us to do so. Just as our body includes pleasure systems that reward us for sex, our brain contains nerve cells that can only be activated by exposure to the molecular structure of THC (The main active ingredient in cannabis). Sex and cannabis provide us with extreme euphoric experiences, a union of body and soul and a healthy escape from routine existence.

Not long ago, the U.S. government prohibited almost all research into the effects of marijuana, now increasingly called cannabis, probably due to the stigma attached to the old name. One welcome consequence of the new wave of legalisation has been an increase in research into its effects—including its impact on lovemaking. Normally, individuals that enjoy cannabis claim that everything tastes, smells and feels that much better when they are high. Dr. Mitch Earleywine, professor of psychology at the State University of New York at Albany explains that "That CB1 receptor seems to be involved in improved tactile sensations and general euphoria." In other words, when this receptor is activated, we get randy.

In a 2009 study by the Australian Research Centre in Sex, women who reported frequent cannabis consumption were also more likely to report more than two sexual partners in the previous year. For men, any cannabis consumption was associated with "a doubling of the likelihood of reporting two or more partners." Stanford researchers found that men who used it weekly reported 22 percent more sex, women 34 percent more. Among those who used cannabis more than weekly, sexual frequency increased even more. This study did not ask if participants found cannabis sex-enhancing, but that can certainly be inferred.

Researchers at St. Louis University in Missouri said that 68 percent said it made sex "more pleasurable," with almost two-thirds (62 percent) saying that it increased their libidos and the pleasure of orgasm. In addition, 16 percent of users reported consuming cannabis prior to sex specifically to relieve pain that interfered with it. Only 3 percent of respondents called the herb sex-killing. Saliva's dominant background is mainly known for its boosting of creativity, and other studies have found that cannabis smokers are more opened to trying new things, especially in bed, and regularly outperform non-smokers.

Background and History

Early western scholars attempting to reconstruct the history of cannabis simply lacked an adequate knowledge of entheogens as a whole. This can be seen in the work of the Viennese Orientalist, Joseph von Hammer-Purgstall who mistakenly regarded hashish and opium as interchangeable terms for the same drug.

One person who actually became acquainted with and studied cannabis use in the Orient was the French physician Jacques Joseph Moreau de Tours. It was he who, in 1843, introduced the revolutionary green paste to the Parisian "Club de Hashischins." Both Gérard de Nerval and Charles Baudelaire were soon writing about its stimulating effects on the imagination and on eroticism. In Baudelaire's words, "Hashish can awaken tender memories in an imagination that is accustomed to occupying itself often with the affairs of love." Eugène Delacroix (1798–1863), the hero of Romantic painters everywhere, was an occasional guest at the hashish meetings and it undoubtedly influenced the vital fire of his colours and orgiastic compositions.

Rudolf Gelpke, a Swiss born Islamic scholar, also noted 'erotic' effects, claiming these effects were due to the fact that it stimulates the imagination. "The more imaginative a person is, and the more his imagination and his sense of the erotic permeate and accentuate one other, the more likely it is that his hashish inebriation will also take on an erotic overtone." In his most famous paper, "On Travels in the Universe of the Soul", he also reported on self experimentation using (LSD) conducted with his friends Dr. Albert Hofmann, and writer Ernst Jünger.

Long before these western observations, Cannabis had been employed as a therapeutic agent by the Ayurveda and Unani Tibbi systems of medicine for millennia. Hindu references to cannabis appear regularly in veterinary and medical works belonging to the twelfth to thirteenth centuries A.D. onwards. Bhavamishra (fifteenth century A.D.), a contemporary of Paracelsus, has in his compendium on medicine and therapeutics, 'Bhavaprakasha,' described the properties, actions, indications and formulations of cannabis.

Even more amazingly, the Ayurvedic system appears to have adopted cannabis from Arabian medicine. The Unani Tibbi system, was brought to India around about the ninth century A.D. by the Muslims, who appear to have recognized cannabis as a therapeutic agent much earlier than Ayurveda did. Arabian medicine came to be known in India as "Unani Tibbi" in view of its Greek origins. Galen of Pergamon (129-201 A.D.) and Rhazes (854-925 A.D.) both gave detailed descriptions of the actions, therapeutics and uses of cannabis. Authoritative Arabic and Persian medical works such as the 'Firdo usul-Hikmat' and the 'Mujardat Quanan' have not only described the properties, but have also included a number of formulations, and potions containing cannabis that were popular in Arabia, Persia and Muslim India. In both systems of medicine, cannabis has been used to produce euphoria, increase libido, conquer potency and cure various diseases. Dozens of formulas containing cannabis have been found to stimulate desire and their names even sound delicious: shrimadananda modaka, utama vajikarana, majun falaskari, roghan bhang. These formulas were thought to improve erectile duration, inhibition of ejaculation and improved lubrication.

In Ayurveda medicine, the treatment that is adopted to increase libido is called "vajikarana," and is used to increase the sexual strength of a man ('Vaaji' translate as Horse in Hindi.) The main aim of Vajikarana therapy is to increase erections, sperm count and sperm mobility. As well as increasing duration of erections, preventing premature ejaculations and erectile dysfunction, it is even claimed that it increases body energy levels and retards the aging process, ensuring that men who undergo this therapy look attractive and never get tired.

The use of cannabis for sexual purposes transcended hedonism and medicine, and was rooted in the esoteric Buddhist tradition known as Tantra, a mystical religion according to which physical and mental exercises such as meditation and yoga were performed. Tantra practitioners believe that the human body contains energy systems that include nerves, heart and spiritual elements linked to cosmic energies and energies of nature. Researchers have discovered sacred texts describing the cults of cannabis who employed advanced tantra rituals designed to help escape suffering and reach a state of enlightenment and perfection, also known as nirvana.

The Tantra rituals used in cannabis were first practiced in the seventh century AD, and involved groups of purified males and females who participated in fasting, sacred poetry, prayer, ritual purification. The Tantra practitioners did not smoke cannabis. Instead, they produced a cannabis drink called Bhang. Sometimes it was nothing more than a green cannabis mixed with milk, but it could also be a delicious milkshake made from selected cannabis leaves and mixed with milk, sugar, pepper, almonds, cardamom, poppy seeds, ginger and other herbs. The mixture was heated before serving to allow THC to reach the form in which it affects humans.

Bhang was known in India as early as the fourth and third centuries B.C. Even in modern India Bhang is considered a holy healing drink that heals diseases, brings good luck, exorcises evil spirits and purifies people of their sins.

In many parts of the country, bhang prepared in the form of a syrup using a recipe very similar to Chai, but sweeter and thicker, is consumed on such festive occasions as Holi and Shivaratri. Bhang is still being sold openly in parts of Rajasthan.

After fasting for at least 24 hours, the Tantra disciples imbibed the Bhang, combined with a deep breath from the stomach and imagination exercises. These exercises were said to release blocked energies, release the muscles, improve blood circulation. As the psychoactive effects of the mixture became clearer, believers entered a state of meditation in which they could repeat their holy vows and pray to Kali, the Indian goddess of Tantra, who embodies the creative forces of women. They would then employ yoga techniques to breathe, meditate and control their muscles to achieve "endless orgasms" without ejaculation. Sacred scriptures describe sexual relations under the influence of cannabis lasting seven or eight hours, until "the night of fire envelops the lovers in the orgasm of the whole body," which then erases the ego.

Yogis, fakirs, sadhus and jangamas (nomadic religious mendicants) have long smoked cannabis as an aid to their meditation, concentration and other religious practices. The Naga Sadhus, Aghoris and Tantric Bhairava sects smoke charas as an integral part of their religious practice. Charas is the Hindustani name given to a hashish form of cannabis which is handmade in the Indian subcontinent and Jamaica. During hand-harvesting, flowering buds are rubbed between the palms of the harvesters' hands, and by the end of the day one has perhaps 8 or 9 grams of charas.

Charas plays an important and often integral role in the culture and ritual of certain sects of the Hindu religion, especially among the Shaivs — the sub-division of Hinduism holding Lord Shiva to be the supreme god (in contrast to Vaishnavs who believe Lord Vishnu is the supreme god)—and it is venerated by some as being one of the aspects of Lord Shiva. It is regaining the popularity it once enjoyed with younger generation of India, regarding it as a recreational drug of choice. It is freely available in several areas around India especially where there is a strong affluence of tourists (Goa, Delhi, Rishikesh, Varanasi, etc.). Although charas can be found in several places around India, its manufacturing can be traced only to specific locations in India such as, Parvati Valley, (Kasol, Rasol, Malana ("Malana cream"), Kashmir as well as several other places in northern India. Tibetans combine leaf powder from young cannabis plants with honey to maintain youth, vitality and sexual potency as well as hair color and texture.

Indian uses of tantra and cannabis are probably the most beautiful and amazing combinations between sexuality and cannabis, but in other cultures there is also the knowledge to use cannabis to improve sexuality. Its use for sexual health has been well documented in Chinese texts, amongst Germanic tribes and by many African cultures.

People's clinics in Serbia of the 19th century relied on a hemp mixture, which was called Nasha. Virgin women received a mixture of lamb fat and cannabis on their wedding night, to relieve the pain of first penetration. This use is similar to the modern use of cannabis in India, where newly married couples drink bhang drinks and eat bananas. Women who work as prostitutes in India tend to eat large amounts of bhang sorbet, which helps them feel sexually aroused even if their clients are ugly and obese.

Serbian women mixed cannabis with egg whites, saffron and sugar to make a tonic that created a sexual mood. These types of tonics that included cannabis were also given to children who used to cry a lot, and it was said that this brought them back to a smiling mood.

Morocco, Egypt, Lebanon and cultures in other countries in the Middle East and North Africa used cannabis for sexual purposes at the beginning of the 20th century. Women and concubines had fun with the servants and used it when the men were not around, and often engaged in erotic fantasies. Cannabis had a reputation for allowing women to become sexually uninhibited, which was a particularly important advantage in cultures where they were routinely suppressed.

The relationship between the Schedule I status of cannabis in the United States and the lack of scientific research has been described as a "catch-22" paradox: cannabis is restricted in large part because there is little research to support medical uses; research is difficult to conduct because of tight restrictions.

Although no one has yet identified the mechanisms that are responsible for the apparent benefit of cannabis as a sexual stimulant, the plant's reputation as a sensory sharpener and an emotion enhancer seems to account for much of the effect. Users report that the effects usually increase sensitivity to temperature, taste, touch, visual stimulation, body, enjoyment of music, creating fantasies and mood. Other common effects include changes in the perception of time that usually lead to a sense that time has slowed or more information is processed and felt.

Cannabis itself is a species of flowering herb that is split into three subspecies: indica, sativa, and ruderalis.

The name indica originally referred to the geographical area in which the plant was grown, now known as Afghanistan. Indica plants are short and stocky, featuring leaves that are broad and "chunky." Sativa plants tend to be taller and skinnier and even be lanky in appearance, with leaves that are thin and pointed. Sativa also grows wild in India, especially in the Himalayan foot-hills and the plains extending from Kashmir in the west and Assam in the east, as well as those of Punjab, Bengal, Rajasthan and Kerala. It also grows extensively on the Chinese side of the Himalayas, especially in the provinces of Yunnan, Sichuan and Guizhou.

The Himalayan foothills are in fact a treasure chest of natural ethenogens and mind-expanding plants, but almost none of these are even acknowledged by what is left of modern Chinese culture. There are around seven hundred species of psychedelic mushrooms alone growing on the slopes of the Chinese Himalayas, not to mention the array of psycho-active lichens, enough to keep Philip K. Dick churning out imaginative alternate futures for centuries to come. Among the less well studied species are the climbers and ivies that creep and crawl over almost bare outcropping in this lush fertile climate. I would be very surprised if there are not at least half a dozen varieties that cooked up, have ayahuasca-like properties or mega-doses of natural DMT. After all the Tibetan Lamas must have had something to inspire all that amazing psychedelic thanka art.

Basically, indicas get you stoned while sativas get you high. Indicas provide what has been called a "body high," while sativas deliver more of a "mind high." Indicas tend to decrease energy and are better for consumption in the evening or at night, after the conclusion of the day's work and activities. Potent indica strains may give some patients what is called "couch lock," a condition in which they become so relaxed that they care barely get up from the sofa. The indica high is often referred to as a "body buzz" and has beneficial properties such as pain relief, in addition to being an effective treatment for insomnia and an anxiolytic, as opposed to sativa's more common reports of a cerebral, creative and energetic high, and even, albeit rarely, comprising hallucinations. Differences in the terpenoid content of the essential oil may account for some of these differences in effect.

On average, indica has higher levels of THC compared to CBD, whereas sativa has lower levels of THC to CBD. However, huge variability exists within either species. The medical interests in cannabis are taking this further, and we will see increasing cultivation trends for more strains developed with CBD-dominant ratios. Unfortunately, sativa plants require longer to grow and yield less medicine (flowers) than indica varieties. This is why indica strains have traditionally dominated those available on the black market, where there is no concern for patient need and the sole focus is profit.

When it comes to aroma, indica strains tend to emit musty, earthy, and skunky odours, while sativas smell sweet, fruity, or spicy. This difference in aroma is the result of terpenes, the molecules within the plant that are cousins to cannabinoids like THC and CBD. While these chemicals provide stunningly pungent odours, their greatest benefit to patients is actually their medicinal efficacy. Myrcene, the most common terpene in cannabis, is known to help patients sleep, battling conditions like anxiety and insomnia. If present in a specific strain in a volume greater than 0.5 percent, the strain is considered an indica. If the amount of myrcene is under one half of one percent, then the strain is deemed a sativa. New strains are constantly being created and many are a compromise that possess the ability to kill pain and fight inflammation while not putting a patient to sleep in the middle of the day.

Cannabis ruderalis is a hardier, low-THC variety grown in the northern Himalayas and southern states of the former Soviet Union, characterized by a more sparse, "weedy" growth. A ruderal species generally refers to any plant that is the first to colonize land after a disturbance removing competition. In permaculture species, this is known as a pioneer species rather than a weed. Cannabis ruderalis is smaller than other species and rarely grows over two feet in height. The other main difference is ruderalis enters the flowering stage based on the maturity of the plant, rather than its light cycle. Cannabis geneticists today refer to this feature as "auto-flowering". This means that when crossed with sativa and indica strains, it produces a plant which flowers automatically and is fully mature in 10 weeks. Ruderalis strains are high in CBD, so they are growing in popularity by some medical cannabis users.

Indicas and sativas do seem to affect orgasms differently, but one is not necessarily better than the other - it is all about what feels best for you.

For many of us, it is sativa all the way for orgasms. When climaxing, it literally draws all of the energy from every part of my body and focuses it on that one intense moment. A sativa helps to pick me up to keep me going, whereas an indica tends to put me into a sex coma. There again, I also notice a lot more mental chatter with sativas than indicas. I want to do everything all at once, whereas the indica I feel relaxed and willing to take my time to really enrich the experience. I also find it much easier to go back for a second orgasm with the indica, whereas after a sativa-enhanced orgasm, I often feel like I want to rewrite 'War and Peace' or eliminate global poverty.

Rather than an either or, it is more about the ratio of THC and CBD. The cannabis plant contains roughly 100 cannabinoids, which are its active components. The best-known of these is THC, which is believed to be mainly responsible for cannabis' psychotropic effects, including cannabis's high. But another cannabinoid, CBD, does not contribute to euphoria and is legal when used recreationally. CBD derived from either hemp or cannabis is legal in 46 states when used medicinally. Some products aimed at improving your sex life contain CBD but not so much THC. These are topical creams, ointments or lubricants that capitalize CBD's apparent anti-inflammatory effects. Too much THC, and I am a heart pounding mess. Micro-dosing with edibles is amazing. 1-3mg of THC evokes just enough of that mental shift. However, it is important to remember that edibles are wildly different per person due to how they are processed in the body.

A high-CBD strain or concentrate before sex can help get you out of your head and into your body, especially for people who cannot or do not want to be high.

The best option is a good mixture of euphoria and relaxation without too much knock-out power. This leads to less anxiety for newer sexual partners, lessening potential erectile difficulties which can stem from anxiety. Because there is so much nuance to cannabis, it is great for those who can, to visit a dispensary and chat with a bud tender who understands cannabinoids and terpenes, and can make recommendations based on the effects you are seeking.

Think about what kind of sex are you want to have? (Solo, partnered, slow lovemaking, frenzied lust, etc.) Think about how your body reacts to different strains and whether different methods of consumption affect you differently. I find that smoking and vaping both affect me in wildly different fashions. If I am tense and feeling anxious, but I want to be in a sexy mood, I might choose something with high CBD to help my body relax and to counteract some of my anxiety. If on the other hand, I am feeling sluggish but want to have really frenzied lustful sex, I might choose something that is more creative and energetic. Remember also that cannabis has a definite entourage effect. This means that the whole plant matters and isolated chemical formulas such as K2, Spice and AK47 can be so unpleasant.

Just a quick note here regarding the word cannabis. Having grown up in the UK, I much prefer this word over marijuana with its unpleasant historical baggage. Words like pot and dope, these are loaded terms that developed huge amounts of stigma during the War on Drugs. Language has an immense sticking power, and we now need to shed the negative stereotypes associated with these terms, especially if we want to educate the general population about its diversity, health and recreational benefits. Therefore, I have used the word cannabis throughout this book to cover all aspects of the wonderful hemp plant, but rest assured, this includes hash, ganja, mary jane and all the other slang terms with which we grew up.

A Growing Choice of Solutions

As cannabis becomes more legal, the industry surrounding it continues to expand. As the much-maligned plant continues to gain the acceptance and recognition that it truly deserves, the popularity of new and innovative products have literally exploded. In San Francisco, which is currently the epicentre of cannabis culture, it seems that every other week there's a local news story about a mom who became a millionaires baking and selling edibles. Whether you are a recreational user seeking the perfect high or you rely on cannabis to manage an illness, there are now dozens of choices on how to consume. You may not be aware of these developments, as prominent search engines like Google are not particularly keen on letting people advertising cannabis products on their website, even if the state it is produced in is legal.

Edibles for example have gone from simple home-made brownies and cookies, to haute cuisine ingredients for gourmets and gastronomes. Cooking with cannabis-infused ingredients has suddenly become a hot new trend for avant-garde chefs and cannabis connoisseurs alike. Cannabis supper clubs are the latest fine-dining trend sweeping Los Angeles and cannabis-infused dining is also on the rise in Canada. Travis Petersen is an Edmonton cannabis chef and owner of The Nomad Cook, who throws "secret" dinners across the country. For $175, each guest (over the age of 19) gets a five-course, cannabis-infused meal, where Petersen micro-doses for every person's tolerance. Alcohol is not served, but they do have CBD-infused mocktails.

Cannabis contains a group of compounds called cannabinoids, one of which is anandamide, also found in chocolate. Anandamide's name derives from the Sanskrit word ananda, which means bliss. In the human brain, anandamide binds to the same receptor sites as THC from cannabis. Anandamide produces a

feeling of euphoria. This compound may account for why some people become blissed-out when they eat chocolate. Not everybody will fall madly in love, become highly sexually aroused, or swoon with ecstatic bliss after a bite of good chocolate. Individual chemistry plays a major role in how people react to chocolate, as it does with almost everything else. Chocolate may produce a modest effect in some people, but it will make others swoon.

Chocolate and cannabis are both a lot like wine. Once you get into them, you discover that fine chocolates offer different flavours and aromas according

to the origin of the beans from which they are made. The same is true for cannabis and even within a small geographic region, varieties can vary widely in their characteristics, due to differences in soil and climate. In the worlds of wine and coffee we have seen a transformation from homogeneous flavours to unique varietals. It used to be that you drank red or white wine. Now you choose a Napa Valley Sauvignon Blanc or a South African Chardonnay. With coffee, you can choose Colombian Supremo, or Kenya AA, or Malaysian Old Town Sugar cane Classic. As people's tastes become more sophisticated, they want to try new flavours. This phenomenon is very clear in the chocolate market and is now occurring in the cannabis sector too.

Newbies going too far above 20-35mg are likely to make

sexual functioning difficult, if not impossible. Start with 5mg if you are a beginner, 10mg if you're a moderate consumer, and for the advanced consumers, I would not go too far about 35-45mg per serving, but do what feels best for your body. Also, be sure to give it time. – Depending on your body chemistry, tolerance, and metabolism, an edible high could last anywhere from 4 to 12+ hours, and that is after the 1-2 hours it takes to kick in. Take deep breaths and drink lots of water. Make sure you are in a safe space where you can properly relax. If possible, have CBD on hand. CBD is great for counteracting a too intense high. If you find yourself in a situation where you have over-consumed (intentionally or not), it is a good idea to have a high CBD strain or vape on hand to help bring you out of the everything-is-overwhelming zone.

Tinctures, oils and balms are all becoming commonplace. Cannabis oil can be taken by itself in a number of different forms. That versatility has made it easily the most sought-after cannabis product for people looking for legal use.

CBD oils have exceedingly low traces of THC, so they will not give you the high that you would normally associate with cannabis. That way one can potentially get the desired effects - pain relief, nausea relief, sexual stimulation etc. - without psychoactive reactions.

Cannabis has been used in pain management for a long time, but over the past few years, ointments and creams infused with THC and CBD have exploded in popularity. They do not all have psychoactive effects, but they do provide serious localized pain relief. Many people, including athletes, have started using these creams instead of reaching for OTC pain relievers because they are great at relieving muscle aches without any of the potential side effects of medication. But CBD oil has also shown itself to be useful with regard to pain relief, cancer treatment, anxiety, depression, and sleep issues, among other conditions. Neuropathic pain patients report relief when used regularly, as well as some who report relief from topical rashes and inflammations. Decarbed cannabis cream works wonders for shingles. Epilepsy is the condition that seems to get the most consistent support for use of cannabis oil, even federally; the U.S. Food and Drug Administration (FDA) recently got a unanimous vote by their federal advisory committee to recommend approval of a pharmaceutical CBD oil known as Epidiolex, which can be used to treat certain rare forms of epilepsy.

Cannabis is slowly becoming a very important ingredient in beauty and skin care products. Many have anti-inflammatory properties due to cannabinoid receptors in skin and can even help fight acne. Hydrating skin oils are specially effective in high altitude areas with high levels of ultra violet and ultra low levels of humidity. Cannabis body wash, lip gloss, and mascara are all being sold on popular related web sites such as Sephora's, while cannabis bubble bath, bath bombs and bath salts can bring some much-needed relief and relaxation in the tub. Exciting research continues on regeneration oils that are combined with other oils such as tea tree oil.

Cannabis tinctures utilize alcohol extraction to remove the THC from cannabis while getting rid of the plant matter. Once extracted, they can be used in a multiplicity of methods. cannabis molasses for example can be substituted anywhere sugar is used. In addition, all kinds of cannabis drinks are slowly making their way to market, from cannabis wine to cannabis vodka and THC-infused cocktails. Kalvara is one of the first to hit the shelves and is currently available in Las Vegas dispensaries. Each 2 oz. serving comes with 10mg of THC that's suspended in nitrogen and instantly infused with the drink once the cap is turned, using a method known as sonic emulsification. It comes in a citrus flavour, does not have to be refrigerated, has a precise THC dosage and appears to have an indefinite shelf life. There are now cannabis-infused non-alcoholic beers in Colorado, while breweries like Coalition Brewing have CBD beer available at select locations in both Oregon and Washington. Beer producers are on the lookout for crossover products and entryways into the growing cannabis industry. While the popularity of craft beer continues to grow across all demographics, alcohol sales continue to decrease in most states, especially where recreational cannabis is available as an alternative. Cannabier helps traditional alcohol-based beer drinkers avoid getting too drunk and later having health problems like liver disease. Plus, most people would rather drink a non-alcohol cannabis infused beverage that ends the day with a good night's sleep rather than vomiting hangovers and the aftermath of a night of bad decision-making. Two Roots cannabis beer recently hit the shelves in Las Vegas and is exclusively sold ReLeaf cannabis dispensary. The THC high hits quicker than most edibles and has a 5 to 10-minute onset time with effects that dissipate after about 90 minutes.

Other manufacturers are working on herbal liqueurs similar to Jagermeister or Chartreuse, but including cannabis in the herb blend used in its preparation. Because of regulatory issues there probably are not many, or any, examples of this on the market in the US yet, but it definitely will not be long. In the meantime, we are seeing an explosion of cannabis colas, sodas and fruit punches. And multiple coffee shops in New York sell cannabis-infused coffees, perfect for calming down anyone who gets the jitters from a strong cup.

We are now seeing lollipops, gum rubs, inhalers, transdermal patches that function similar to a nicotine patch, and even CBD-infused chewing gum

Cannabis pizzas and shakes have long been popular on the backpacker circuit in Asia, and can be found everywhere from Tiger Leaping Gorge, to Angkor Wat and all the way down to beaches of Bali. Americans are now starting to experiment with canna milks and canna ice creams, and it probably will not be long before Ben and Jerry have a 'Spoonful of Loving' cannabis infused flavour. Of course, the simplest and safest way to consume cannabis is to just break off a piece of decarboxylated bud and eat it. No effort and no waste.

Dr. Mahmoud A. El Sohly, who is in charge of the University of Mississippi's cannabis farm is a famous proponent of the cannabis suppository, also known as the booty bump. When a drug is taken orally and absorbed from the gastrointestinal tract, it enters the portal vein and is metabolised in the liver. If it is one which is principally broken down in the liver-for example, morphine, hydralazine, or propranolol, it does not achieve its optimal effect when taken orally. If it is given through the rectum however, better absorption and greater systemic effect may be achieved. I will talk more about these and other tantric tinctures in the 'Products' chapter.

For Ladies

Throughout history, female deities have been portrayed as electrifying sexual creatures. Religions with sacred cannabis use recognise the metaphysical potential of the female cannabis plant and often portray it as a goddess. Tantric Kali cults such as the Kaula and Krama had a strong influence on Tantric Buddhism, as can be seen in fierce looking yoginis and dakinis such as Vajrayogini and "Krodikali". Other similar fierce deities include the dark blue Ugra Tara and the lion-faced Simhamukha. Because cannabis is so often associated with divine female characters, you can say that when you use cannabis for sexual purposes, you are putting a very special 'woman' into your bed. You need to make sure you are sufficiently prepared for such an experience.

The Tibetan art of sexual ecstasy goes back to the early 8th century, when the beautiful Yeshe Tsogyal, an enlightened consort of Buddha Padmasambhava, was called the "Great Skydancer." Together they developed Tantric sex techniques of the Tibetan masters. Skydancers in the Buddhist tradition were lovers of great passion who were profoundly devoted to spiritual awakening. A new sexual experience in which physical pleasure becomes a delight of the heart and an ecstasy of the spirit. In Tantric Buddhist art, fierce female deities are presented as terrifying, demonic looking beings adorned with human skulls and other ornaments associated with the charnel ground, as well as being often depicted with sexually suggestive attributes. Dakini Demonesses are often portrayed standing over the body of prone male. In south-east Asian traditions, English translations of the word "apsara" include "nymph", "fairy", "celestial nymph", and "celestial maiden". Beautifully adorning the monuments at Angkor Wat, Apsaras are said to be able to change their shape at will, and rule over the fortunes of gaming and gambling. In practically every culture, nymphs are immortal creatures of great beauty and fine bearing. These Houri, also known as muses, artemisians, and nineveh, are always highly fetching creatures of elven wit and fey grace. Modern society so often portrays women as victims and servants when in fact they are vixens, enchantresses and supreme seductress.

One of the most influential women in this rapidly growing area is "cannasexual" Ashley Manta, a professional sex educator whose workshops help people combine cannabis and sex. The reality is that most bud tenders don't know how to talk to their patients about sex, and most sex educators don't know how to talk to their clients about cannabis, and so Ashley has found a unique niche. Much of her work involves dispersing myths about the effects of getting high. Using cannabis does not have to mean getting high at all. There are multiple non-psychoactive methods of consumption, it is just that most people are unfamiliar with them. She receives a large amount of push back from women especially, who have demanding children and cannot commit to being high all day or who simply do not like the feeling of being high. These are both understandable concerns that can be assuaged with topicals, bath soaks, and other products that offer benefits of cannabis without the psychoactive effects.

It is now possible to combine sex and weed without having to get completely wasted. Enjoying cannabis no longer means taking massive bong rips or eating brownies that leave you flying for the next four hours. The application of cannabis oil is a great way to get just your vagina high, a super sexual body high that does not involve having to feel super stoned.

An interesting side effects is that cannabis has a profoundly positive impact on the way that many women feel about their bodies. They are less likely to get caught in the non-stop "you're not pretty/then/flexible enough" narratives by using cannabis to quiet those voices. In fact, cannabis can help to re frame those types of limiting beliefs that the cosmetics industry uses to make women hate their bodies. For example, choose a cannabis product that will help you to relax and make your body feel good then do some exercises where you look in the mirror and say neutral nice things about your body. This works especially well at a dance studio where there are full length mirrors covering all the walls. By the look of all the beaming smiles, I am sure that I am not the only person under the influence at my local weekly Salsa class.

You do not need to get so stoned that you "forget" the things you dislike about your body. This is about mindfully choosing cannabinoid and terpene profiles that will augment the positive changes that you are setting in motion.

In modern-day practical terms, as well as being a super effective arouser, cannabis also functions as a vaginal health supplement by reducing vaginal dryness, which in itself, is one of the leading factors in contracting urinary tract infections (UTIs) and yeast infections. The vaginal walls have a very fragile PH and cannabis oil is extremely effective in ensuring that all the natural systems are fully activated. This solution also avoids the need for broad spectrum antibiotics which are used to combat vaginal infections. Some women prefer to enjoy the physical benefits of vaginal wellness without having the psycho-active side effects and cannabis oil offers both heightened sensation and heightened pleasure.

In terms of sexual health, cannabis can help regulate many

things in the body, like your mood, or pain management due to its interaction with the endocannabinoid system. If you usually feel pain with penetration, then you will definitely notice feeling a more profound level of comfort and similar improvements on blood flow and lubrication. For women that have already reached menopause and often feel that sex is painful due to dryness, using a cannabis oil can be a real relief. It can even increase egg ovulation when oestrogen is at its highest levels. There are not as yet as many studies done for women than men. The female body does, in fact, act differently depending on the oestrogens levels. According to a research done by Professor Rebecca Craft of Washington State University, male rats retraction to cannabis was less sensitive than female rats. As the legalisation process continues, we may find that cannabis has a much more significant impact on women than it does men. For example did you know that the female breast slips naturally produced endocannabinoids into the milk after pregnancy. Note the root cannabis in there. These substances, which cause the munchies, probably play a role in enticing infants to eat. But they also regulate appetite so infants feel very full by the end of a feed and thus do not eat too much. Interestingly, formula lacks these compounds, and formula-fed babies have a notoriously higher caloric intake. It is one of the speculations about why we have a childhood obesity epidemic.

Cannabis is also useful because it facilitates relaxation and mindfulness, two key components of pleasurable sensation. Wetter is always better. You want to be feeling a bit more loosey goosey down there. Completely tension free, like your vagina was kicking back on the beach in Phuket, without a care in the world. Like your pussy had just popped a quaalude and washed it down with a stiff single malt. If you know that you are prone to getting stuck in your head, try a high CBD strain for anxiety. For those who want to amplify sensation, try a strain that makes you extra sensitive to tactile stimuli.

Some studies reveal stereotypical differences between the sexes: women tend to be more conservative than men in their use of cannabis to improve sexual pleasure, and the inability to give up control and enjoy increased sexual stimuli induced by drugs. Each of us has a collection of psychological parameters that determine the effect of cannabis on our sexual desire and pleasure, for better or for worse. Another woman said she was afraid of cannabis because it made her "have sex only for pleasure instead of a normal relationship." Male and female attitudes towards sex are very different. There is an old joke that women need a reason to have sex, while men only require the opportunity.

Men are hungry hedonists and enjoy sex for much the same reasons that theta they enjoy getting high. Women on the other hand tend to have sex for many other reasons. Sometimes, perhaps due to social stigma, it is hard for them to do it just because it feels good. Cannabis can help them to become more liberated with regard to coital concerns. Once they realise that they are indeed a talented lover, even someone they have only just met, can help them achieve orgasm now that they are willing to open themselves up to the idea of pleasure for pleasures sake. Previously, many were told they had to be loved and committed to a relationship so that sex would be respectable and wonderful. Cannabis can stimulate them to the point where they are no longer influenced by outdated religious dogma and social stereotypes.

It is also important to know that an orgasm is simply an involuntary release of muscle tension. For instance, in order to have a stimulation-based orgasm, some women need to be lying down with their legs straight out and clenched. There are many women out there who literally cannot get off if their legs are bent or not flexed. Conversely, some find the tension distracting or interfering with their pleasure due to muscle cramps or the position they need to be in to facilitate orgasm. Experiment with muscle use to find out what works best for you and how you too can achieve total body orgasm and multiple orgasms.

Once women begin to appreciate their own pleasure, they obviously also become better sexual partners. Women who feel more naturally lubricated for example are better to contract the vaginal muscles, increasing the pleasure that they are able to give to a male lover. Remember ladies, that penises are like puppies. They are always so glad to see you but they respond poorly to commands, and the more aggressive you get with your commands, the more they will just cower and wait for you to calm down.

About one in three women find it very difficult to orgasm during sex. Cannabis has the power to make your orgasmic experience unbelievably mind-blowing. We are talking really, really intense, earth-shattering, life-altering orgasms. The kind of ultra-intense orgasms where you find yourself hitting octaves that you had no idea you could reach. Because cannabis has a strange time dilation effect, it will also strengthen your sexual stamina and lengthen your orgasms. Time will appear to move much more slowly and your orgasms will go from lasting thirty seconds, to much, much longer, as well as being incredibly intense.

If you have the chance to be alone, take the time to really sit with and process your physical feelings, without being distracted by all the exciting things that are happening when you are hooking up with someone. When you do finally bring yourself to

35

climax, that concentrated, increased awareness of every nerve in and around your vagina will likely result in an impressive orgasm.

The more we understand our own sexuality and desires, the more we can teach our partners, and the more we can get what we want. To this end, the Lioness is a smart vibrator akin to the Fitbit that tracks a range of usage metrics to give you knowledge of your own arousal and become a true orgasm scientist. Knowledge is power, especially when it comes to sex.

The Lioness is a nicely made vibrator, with a movable head to stimulate the clitoris at the top and an insertable one that reaches deep into the vagina, making orgasms more intense. It also houses biofeedback sensors on the dildo end, which detects pelvic floor and wall contractions. There is another sensor that recognizes when a session starts, by measuring body temperature, which tends to rise as people get aroused. The device also houses an accelerometer and gyroscope to track its motion. This data is displayed in the free Lioness app, on a chart showing waves cresting and falling as the pelvic floor moves. You can see your vaginal contractions represented as spikes or as a circle that contracts and expands.

The vibrator cannot tell if she achieved orgasm, or how strong it was, so you can also record subjective information, writing notes for each climax, making the app a sort of masturbation diary without any real work on your part. You can also tag each session with anything from "five-star" to "drunk" and learn how different outside circumstances impact your sex life. This will give anyone with a vagina a good idea of what their orgasms look like and how long they take to achieve orgasm. It is hoped that the Lioness will hopefully soon be able what type of orgasm you have. One beta tester learned she had a harder time coming when she was menstruating and an easier time coming when ovulating.

While several app-connected vibrators have hit the market in recent years, the Lioness appears to be one of the first to take more ambitious "smart" ideas and actually bring them to market. It is certainly way ahead of all the models manufactured by Chinese companies who sell your most personal data to the highest bidder. There will be a temptation for some companies to gamify this for clueless guys, so that they can say stuff like "I got her to level 23 last night," very proudly. I think that this will be a mistake. We do not want women to come with a technical manual like a car? With each woman being different in what brings her best to orgasm, it has always involved a lot of experimentation and exploration, which lets be honest, is half the fun. Besides, chemistry is dynamic and unique to every couple so what may work for one pairing may not work with the next partner.

Orgasm results from a complex combination of frequency, amplitude, and other measures, but a full scientific understanding of orgasm, particularly clitoral and vaginal orgasms, is still lacking and so the best potential for technologies like Lioness, though, is when all the data is put together.

As long as the data is fully anonymized and permission is obtained before sending it to the cloud, this could be the data source for one heck of a crowd sourced study on female sexuality using data-centric, objective analysis. The fact that it has already introduced us to the concept of orgasm patterns—something about which nothing had been published before—is very promising. Imagine masturbating for the benefit of modern science. I can see onslaught of vagina's posting orgasm diagrams on social media now. At least pussy patterns will be more interesting that endless cat videos.

Lioness is a female-led company that was started by a group of grads at the University of California at Berkeley. The company raised $1.4 million from Creative Ventures and early stage angels, and it debuted the Lioness Vibrator in August 2017. The Lioness initially shipped to Indiegogo crowd-funders before going on sale via the Lioness website. Lioness co-founder and VP of engineering Anna Lee was previously a mechanical design engineer on the Amazon Lab126's Concept Engineering team, and I am sure that she will hate me for saying this, but it has often been the image of her sexy, short haircut that has helped me achieve some of the highest peaks and spikes ever. At $230 it is not cheap, but the world's smartest rabbit vibrator should be seen as a personal health investment. I am hoping for an upgrade with warming option and rechargeable battery, and maybe even a Bluetooth speaker to play some Barry White tracks in the background.

For Gentlemen

The effects of cannabis lubrication oil is just as effective on the male genitals as it is on those of females, and the enhanced cannabis experience is just as cosmic for men as it is for women. The already super-sensitive areas of the glans, the frenum and the perineum are activated to extraordinary levels that you previously would not have thought possible. The flesh inside the foreskin of uncircumcised or intact penises is the same kind of mucous membrane found inside the vulva and rectum, which makes them very susceptible to the sexually enhancing effects of cannabis oils. For those who are circumcised, sadly this is no longer the case.

Most men are socialized to believe that sex involves penetration of an erect penis into some sort of opening (mouth, vagina, or anus). They typically view sex as goal-oriented, performance-driven, orgasm-centric, and erection focused.

This limiting belief can severely impact anybody's ability to enjoy the sex they are having, because they get stuck trying to have the sex they see in porn or movies. The negative impact of porn can be seen most clearly in the growing popularity of Asian ladyboys, rake thin, heavily surgically enhanced and plastered in make up. Only female porn stars, rather than ordinary females resemble these media stereotype and so heavy porn users are unconsciously drawn to these mixed-gender mutants.

It does not help that the recent emergence of the 'pick-up artist' community and the internet 'manosphere' seems to focus much more of quantity than it does on quality. Even since the release of the book, 'The Game' most men seemed to be obsessed with physical appearance and racking up as many conquests as possible as if sex is some kind of high scoring video game. In reality, sex is something to be savoured, a pleasure to be explored and experimented with. The few studies that mention cannabis and sex that the drug's sense of pleasure increases because it increases the sense of touch and the creation of fantasies. Exploring the body with toys, hands, fingers, and tongues, can allow us to see penises (and, more broadly, the genitals) as just another pleasurable place to explore, rather than focusing on them as the main event. Unfortunately most men are still to busy focussing on pick-up lines rather than tantric technique. Very few for example, seem to realise that there is a very physical correlation between a woman's bottom lip and her vagina. If a puckered pout is properly pleasured with some gentle sucking, then the lower lips will puff up accordingly.

Many guys have reported that their erections were bigger and harder when they were stoned, and cannabis is now being used to treat erectile difficulties in men with high cholesterol. Who does not want to last longer in bed? You too can become the superman of sexual partners when you introduce cannabis into the picture. That being said, adding a cock ring to your sexual toolbox will fix any performance problems far more effectively than cannabis alone. Cock rings are applied (with lube!) when the penis is flaccid. As the blood starts to flow in, the ring prevents it from flowing back out, facilitating an erection. The cock ring should go around the shaft and behind the testicles, so that the scrotum and penis are both pulled through it. This ensures pressure is placed on the artery that allows blood to flow back out of the penis. Many seasoned cock ring users report that having blood concentrated in the area enhances sensation and the application of a good quality oil will certainly enhance this feeling. Just be careful not to leave it on when you fall asleep and take it off every 90 minutes or so. Do not let the blood pool nor stagnate or it is a trip to the ER!

If you wish to share your love of cannabis with a new partner, then try starting off by offering a relaxing foot massage. This is far more preferable to immediately offering them a lung-bursting rip from your 5-foot monster bong, especially if they are even slightly asthmatic. Have a discreet vape pen on hand, so as not to give the impression that you think the 'Tao of Steve" is a sacred document, and that you regularly hit the bong before breakfast. In addition, your place should offer an environment that feels both comfortable and can set a seductive mood. After more than thirty years in the odour control business, OMI Industries now offers a Cannabolish line of products for users who don't want their clothes, homes, or cars to smell like smoke. Rather than that funky, fake fragrance of patchouli on top of cannabis odour, the company has developed a formulation that completely eliminates the odour molecule from cannabis and tobacco smoke. A soy-based candle with a 30-hour burn time is destined to become a fixture in dorm rooms around the country. The candle has to warm up, but the oils actually vaporize off of that and into the air, while the spray form is immediate odour control.

Cannabis will affect your perception of time, so try incorporating a few techniques that slow things down into your sexual repertoire as these will definitely increase both your levels of pleasure. For example, take your time undressing each other. Up the ante by making her stand naked with both hands on the edge of the bed and wait for you to undress before taking her from behind. Take your time, as build-up and anticipation are everything.

Whenever you thrust deep inside, pause, and, using your pelvic floor muscles, make your penis "beat" (like a heartbeat) inside of her. Most women have never experienced anything like this before and will usually be impressed. When you eventually come to actual penetration, ask your partner just how bad she wants it, preferably while you have just the very tip inside her. Tell her that she will have to countdown out loud, from ten to zero, and once she reaches lift-off, she will finally have you all the way inside her. Once she begins counting down, just very slightly move your tip as if you were going to thrust all the way in, but go very shallow. With each count she will breathe heavier and start counting a bit louder, like she is getting ready to bungee jump off a cliff-top or leap out of an air-plane. If you are both high, then the audible effects will be that much more impressive.

She will be expecting you to thrust really deep on zero and so will her entire body. The key here is teasing and unpredictability. Try continuing the really shallow thrusting even when she reaches zero and tell her that she is going to have to start counting all over again because the sight of her amazing (insert her best feature here) distracted you and you forgot to go all the way in. Even if she seems frustrated, she will love it really.

She starts counting again, but this time you are going to surprise her. When she hits 3 Or 2, ram inside her all the way really hard and really fast. The sound she makes at this point varies from woman to woman, and can vary from high pitch squealing, to full-on scream-queen being chopped up by an axe murderer. Do not be surprised if one of your neighbours calls the police. Just one deep thrust has a very immediate impact, but you can also jack hammer her into oblivion for much faster orgasm that she will remember for the rest of her life. It all varies according to you and that is why it is so fun. The next time you use the trick (and you can use it again and again), she will be guessing what "number" she will get it at. Chances are that once you tell her to start counting, she will say 10, 9,...zero! Get it in! Make her count all the way anyway. This incredible amount of unpredictability is definitely one of the things women love in bed. From then on, you will always be the guy who did that thing to her with the counting that she loved so much.

Continuing with the theme of uncertainty and unexpectedness. Innovation is a valuable in the bedroom as it is anywhere. Pillow fights and naked wrestling are a great way to recreate the passion and sexy romp you get with make up sex. A little play-fighting will get you both "up and at 'em." Mild bondage heightens sexual urgency. Use simple household items, like the belt off a silk robe, to tie each other up. Take this one step further by "going caveman" on her. Literally rip her panties off, just make sure it is not a pair of expensive VS undies that she wore specially for the occasion. If you have never ripped a woman's panties off, you cannot really say that you have lived. Stick your fingers in her pussy, then shove them in her own mouth and make her suck on them while you resume fucking her.

Toy with her so that she knows she is about to get either slapped or bitten... but she does not know when, building up the anticipation. Slap her ass three times, then jerk your hand like you are about to slap it again, but do not actually do it! Fake her out, then fake her out again, and finally when she is not expecting it, slap her ass super hard. Do the same thing with biting her neck. Randomly bite it super-fast while you are kissing, sometimes hard and sometimes soft. Bite her, pull her hair and generally fuck her like a caveman. Even hair pulling has a technique. Place your open hand on the back of her neck and then insert your fingers into her hair. This way you will have hold of a good mass of hair and can yank her head back, without causing any real pain. There is nothing more painful than a careless guy yanking a small strand of hairs. Make love in random semi-public place, like in your car in an empty parking lot at night or by the bedroom window with the blinds open. Again this adds to the excitability.

Many of the Boomers who were smoking pot when today's Millennials were still a gleam in their parents' eyes are now some of the oldest members of society and may not be up to rigours of the modern single's scene. There is a serious misconception that human beings have an expiration date when it comes to sexual expression and sexual pleasure. This is not true, and we are all lifelong sexual beings. Even so, pain and pain avoidance become ever more important issues as our continually aging bodies begin to challenge our active lives. Specially formulated products like the extra-strength pain spray, Apothecanna, is highly recommended for relief of arthritis and joint pain. After all, nobody wants to feel like they are a creaky old coffin dodger that might snap at any moment when they are getting frisky. As the stigma of doing something shady and illegal is reduced, seniors can also benefit from the increased sensation and relaxation and decreased pain during sex. This will in turn increase the frequency of sex simply because it would be so pleasurable again, creating a wonderfully virtuous circle.

Of course, there is no need to go without just because you do not currently have a partner. People who enjoy cannabis alone can also have sex with themselves. Try it on your own first. You don't know what effects a product or strain will have on your body before trying it since everyone is different, so it's important to test things out on your own so you know the effects in advance. One innovative suggestion is to create your very own pleasure map. Cannabis affects all of our bodies very differently depending on tolerance, strain, and method of consumption. So once you are feeling the effects, take time to explore your entire body. Cannabis can bring nerve endings on-line in a powerful way, and you will never know which ones you might have missed and how you like to be stimulated, unless you experiment. Afterwards, reflect on how you have felt in different places on different strains and you will have a better and more detailed understanding of how the different varieties of cannabis can impact your sex life. I suggest taking the time with a new product or strain to enjoy it, notice the effects it has on your body, then masturbate and notice those effects too. That way when you use it with a partner, you can isolate variables more readily if something is not feeling quite right. Many guys report that orgasm can feel even stronger if they happen shortly after a good, strong bowel movement. Although I am not a doctor, this does actually make sense, as the prostate is situated in that region of the body and is very susceptible to differences in pressure. The effect of a good cannabis lube on a prostate massage would very likely be little short of cataclysmic. Although most lubes and tinctures have been created to amplify sexual pleasure in females, and is marketed toward vaginal use, the majority are also safe to eat and, if you are brave enough to put up your butt. If you would like to give the not-so-gentle art of pegging a try, then a cannabis lubricant would be a very useful facilitator.

So, far there has been very little research on the effects that cannabis has on gay male sex, but there is plenty of highly positive anecdotal research. A number of single sex pairings have tried spray lubes, using between four and eight pumps generously to a dildo - one pump on, insert gently, then another pump, and so on. Initial reports state that it makes 'bottoming' extremely easy, plus there are no poppers headaches or accidentally spilled chemicals, and less room for error in the heat of the moment, when it really counts. Gay guys will still want to use regular lube. Although cannabis oils are sold as stimulation lubes, and they do work as such, they may not reduce friction enough to facilitate gay anal sex, which requires tons of lube to work. This might also be good advice for mixed pairing peggers. As we continue to explore the boundaries between drug use and sexuality, cannabis lube will redefine the way we think about stimulants and our bodies. And, in the end, it will produce some wicked good sex, no matter where you are putting what.

For those of you who are still afraid of anal penetration, a more acceptable alternative might be the ballcuzzi. Take a warm bowl of water and sprinkle in some Epsom salts. In North America you will also be able to find some cannabis infused bath salts, such as those in the Whoopi and Maya line. Gently dip your testicles in the water and have your partner female to blow bubbles in the water with a straw while she stimulates you manually. You will be amazed at how awesome this feels, like a luxury spa for your testicles.

For Lovers

Nothing creates a deeper and more meaningful relationship than shared sexual bliss. If you can transform the sex act from being a chore that a woman feels she has to perform to please her man, to being a mind-blowing experience that they never dreamed possible. With cannabis as a spiritual and physical enhancer, you will be able to create a connection that is far deeper than 99% of other couples ever come close to achieving.

It is always a good idea to try using cannabis solo before bringing in a partner, but sometimes idea of doing it together for the first time is part of the appeal.

Negotiating before medicating is especially applicable to new partners. Have a conversation about safer sex needs and what is on the menu for sexy fun time activities. Start with a bottle of infused oil for massage. It is a great way to get things started, and it can feel a lot safer for new users to enjoy the somatic benefits of cannabis without the head high. Sex with cannabis is way more intense, intimate and connected. It can be incredibly intimate, and once you have established that you both enjoy the experience, then you can move onto other methods of consumption. In time, you can think about taking a bath together using a cannabis infused bath bomb, (while drinking cannabis infused wine obviously) and finishing off with some infused cannabis ice cream. Advanced couples might want to contrast the intense romanticism of the evening by following up with a frenzied pegging session, utilising cannabis lube, of course.

Contrary to the myth of reefer madness, according to which cannabis automatically leads to uncontrollable sexual desire, cannabis and sexuality have been closely linked to each other for thousands of years. Long traditions of sacred sexuality and sexual mysticism connect the spiritual practices of India, Tibet, Nepal, China, Mongolia, and Japan. Inspired by the classical teachings of the tantric texts, western sexual mysticism is currently enjoying a renaissance. Yoga teachers discovering the sexual dimensions of their craft have reconstructed the tantra that birthed it. The iconoclastic guru Osho (Bhagwan Shree Rajneesh) developed and taught his own understanding of tantra, which gave birth to what is often called 'neotantra.' Other teachers, perhaps most notably David Deida, are starting with tantric principles as a foundation for their own unique lines of teaching. In some of these teachings, the relevance and role of sexuality is the very heart of the teaching.

In Indian legend, the Hindu goddess Parvati was annoyed that her husband Shiva was such a philanderer, and decided to do something about it. When Shiva returned home, she gave him hemp leaves, which Shiva smoked for the first time in cosmic history. Not only did it make him feel happy and aroused, but it opened his third eye, and he realized that the divine Parvati was the most beautiful being in the universe. People today still smoke ganja to honour Shiva today. There is a Shivaratri in every luni-solar month of the Hindu calendar, on the month's 13th night/14th day, and once a year in late winter (February/March), marks Maha Shivaratri which means 'The Great Night of Shiva.' If cannabis were legal worldwide, maybe this annual celebration could become a global divorce reconciliation event.

There is some debate among stuffy academic circles as to the prevalence and importance of sexuality in the teachings of embodied mindfulness and in the rituals of classical tantra. But it was undoubtedly present. One manual teaches the discovery of unity with the divine in the bliss of orgasm. In another case, one of the most influential teachers of the Krama lineage, Cakrabhānu, was imprisoned and branded for corrupting the Brahmin class of his town with his licentious rituals.

The temple architecture of Vajrayana Buddhism in Khajurao, a direct descendent of tantric teaching, is vivid with imagery of the lingam (penis), the yoni (vulva & vagina), and deities locked in carnal embrace. Illustrations from the tantric tradition glorify both practitioner and consort in sexual union. It is often assumed that the male is the practitioner and the female is the consort, but this is increasingly seen as a misunderstanding. Men and women were equal practitioners in tantra, and the great teachers were often female (although the great writers were often male).

Classical tantra largely died out in the 1100s. Islam arrived in India. Buddhism retreated, and tantric practice largely disappeared. Eight to nine hundred years later, Tantra has sprung back to life, with all the diversity, vibrancy, and ferment of its early blossoming.

Modern users report spiritual, emotional, and psychological effects that were very similar to the effects described in Tantra. Influenced by cannabis, they felt that sexual intercourse was an activity of energy exchange that united the bodies in a cosmic circle. They felt that the exchange was refreshing and balanced, and that the orgasm was the energetic climax. For both sexes, orgasms are likely to be felt throughout the body, not just in the genital area. Users engaged in sexual activity are more aware of the signs leading to orgasm and were more free to perform body movements that increased the pleasure.

Some users report that sex combined with cannabis opened the doors of perception. It lifted them beyond the ego into spiritual worlds where sexual activity was of symbolic and universal importance. Many also noted that it seems that cannabis helped them feel more loving towards their partners. Cannabis users who have experienced yoga and meditation felt that cannabis increased their self-awareness of their internal organs and more delicate internal processes in their bodies.

When the dose is appropriate, users report that it increased their ability and duration of the activity, the sensation, duration and intensity of the orgasms, and even the psychic connection between the partners. People felt they were more willing to pay more attention to the technical aspects of making love and the preliminary foreplay, something that most women complain of is usually lacking in the repertoire of male sexual activities. In contrast, women report that their lovers were all of a sudden surprisingly skilled. Everything their partners did felt good — there was no shuffling to find the exact right spot because everything felt like the right spot.

Cannabis encourages bonding, and it is well-known that smoking alone is not as fun as smoking with someone else. Studies have found that couples who smoke together have less aggression, and are much less prone to violence towards each other. Having a similar interest contributes to having a healthier relationship, and a healthier sex life. I certainly find myself more deeply connected and more energetically open when I consume with a partner. Little empirical data on this phenomenon exists, but studies have shown that the endocannabinoid system can stimulate the production of oxytocin. A hormone produced in the hypothalamus and distributed by the pituitary gland, oxytocin is widely known as the "bonding hormone." And according to The Washington Post, the University of Buffalo studied over 600 couples ranging as far back as 1996 and found that couples who smoke weed really do fight less.

If you both enjoy oils, edibles and other forms of cannabis, then why not try to more traditional methods of smoking together. After all, it does seem based on the evidence that couples who blaze together, stay together. Rolling a joint can be surprisingly therapeutic for many people, and the feeling of doing something that has long been portrayed in the movies as naughty and illicit can add that little extra frisson to any relationship. Start with one puff or one hit of a vape. Inhalation effects set in pretty quickly, so you will only need to wait 10-15 minutes before deciding if you want more. Try smoking a body-heavy indica strain like GDP or Northern Lights and spend time holding and cuddling with your partner with no specific agenda — just enjoy touching and caressing. Pairing cuddling with some deep eye gazing, is one of my favourite techniques for enhancing intimacy and adding add a deeper level of connection. Lay on a flat, comfortable surface facing one another. Get as close as possible, literally belly to belly, and wrap your arms around each other. Then you gaze into the left eye of your partner. In tantra, the left eye is considered the receptive eye. Do it for as long as it feels comfortable (try 1-2 minutes at first), and notice what you find there. Many people report feeling more deeply connected with their partner after this exercise. Do not be caught up in the misunderstanding that tantric sex involves impossible feats of bodily contortionism and superhuman flexibility. Tantra is often surprisingly simple.

If you prefer the effects of more cerebral sativa strains, then try to find bedroom activities that are equally stimulating. You do not want a variety that makes you rambling, incoherent, and tangential, so try by it out by yourself first to get a good idea of the effects. You definitely do not want a strain that turns you into a classical philosopher, nor do you want something that makes it a challenge to string more than a few words together.

Practicing solo creates new neural pathways that make it easier to default to new behaviours. This way you can notice what sensations arise in your body while masturbating. Narrating what is going on in your body is a great baseline for talking dirty with a partner and you can always come back to that, because you know what is happening in your body if you tune into it. Another effective method is to buy a book of erotica and two highlighters in different colours. Each partner goes through and highlights all the passages that turn them on. This way you will have amazing first-hand data on what kinds of words and phrases turn on your partner, and it is also a great way to see where your interests overlap. Always try to stay hydrated. Dry mouth is a common side effect of consuming cannabis, especially when smoking, and it can be a real challenge to make words happen when your mouth feels like the Taklamakan Desert.

Cannabis is well-known for its inhibition-reduction effects, so if you have never tried masturbating in front of a partner, this is a good chance. Showing your partner how you like to be touched can be a powerful tool for hotter sex. Do not just give a silent demonstration, explain what it feels like to stimulate these areas, and it will help you become more comfortable communicating your pleasure preferences.

One especially innovative idea is to integrate the creation of art into your sex life. The 'Love is Art Kit' has been created by abstract artist Jeremy Brown, but you can easily make your own. All you need is a large plastic drop cloth, a slightly smaller canvas, some non-toxic paint, and a couple of pairs of disposable slippers so you do not track paint on the floor afterwards, when heading for the shower. You will then be able to immortalize one magical night into an art form, and create a masterpiece that you will both be able look at and recall your time together with fondness and love. Start off with a couple of cannabis chocolate edibles, a couple of joints or your favourite massage oil while setting up your play space. Move any unnecessary furniture out of the way and tape down the corners of the tarp and canvas so that your vigorous lovemaking will not cause it to bunch up. Jeremy Brown recommends setting up candles in the shower beforehand, so you can continue the experience as you rinse off. His directions also suggest starting sexy fun times off on the couch, then moving to the canvas and applying the paint once everyone was sufficiently warmed up. It is also a good idea to place the paint bottles in warm water so that they are warmed up too. Having sex while simultaneously using your body as a paintbrush is a unique and hilarious experience. This is a fun and artistic way to immortalize any relationship.

If you are looking for more inspiration on indulgent sex play, I highly recommend the book 'Fifty Shades of Sexual Fantasy' by my fellow author Darby Jones. Inside its pages, you will discover fifty exquisite, sensuous fantasies that will transform your sex life into a series of exotic adventures that would have made even Casanova and Madame de Pompadour green with envy.

Not all erotic encounters need to be enjoyed at home. Many cannabis enthusiasts report increased appreciation of aesthetics when high, so why not take a stroll in the park, watch the sunset over the sea, or hike to a high-altitude lookout with sweeping views. The feeling of the wind sweeping through your hair and the beauty of the stars makes for a truly magical nature experience.

Whatever you get up to, you can certainly look forward to a good deep sleep afterwards. Both sex and cannabis are both natural insomnia cures, and together they have a very powerful synergistic effect.

Canna Erotica

A growing number of entrepreneurial twenty-somethings are riding a wave of marijuana legalization to make a living getting stoned on YouTube. These weed-centric YouTubers – or WeedTubers, as they call themselves are the Cheech and Chong for the digital age. They may not be millionaires like some YouTube stars, but WeedTube's irrefutable king, Joel Hradecky, whose channel, CustomGrow420, has amassed a following of more than 1.2 million since 2013. A video in which he tries to smoke a gram of THC oil has racked up more than 1.3m views. A subsequent video of him coughing for nearly seven minutes straight after the attempt has more than 1.5m views. Many viewers want to see feats of consumption they would never dare try themselves – smoking an entire gram of cannabis in one minute, for instance – and, of course, the grisly aftermaths. People obviously like watching other people suffer. As an influential cannabis connoisseur, Hradecky is paid between $300 and $1,000 per video to promote bongs, marijuana strains and other accessories on his channels, plus money for every new customer they refer. Once cannabis is re legalised around the world, it will be normalised and eventually these channel's popularity will fade.

In the meantime, even more popular are the female WeedTubers who post videos of themselves on Periscope in weed-printed bikinis or booty shorts, or even doing bong rips naked. Within the cannabis industry, the image of women who regularly smoke weed is fairly one-dimensional. Women have been hired as booth babes and to sell bongs for decades. Thanks to Instagram accounts for apparel companies like Bong Beauties and scantily clad models on the covers of publications like High Times, women within the marijuana industry have traditionally been heavily sexualized, relegated to the role of short-skirted "dab tender" at cannabis expos. Culturally speaking, the trope of the female pot smoker is a relatively new one, but thanks to shows like Broad City and celebrities like Rihanna, the image of the laid-back, sexy female stoner is rapidly gaining prominence in popular culture.

It is not uncommon to see women on Periscope taking naked bong hits or showing extensive cleavage, presumably as a way to cater to their predominantly male audience. A quick search for #weedporn on Instagram will turn up nearly seven million images, but these are mostly superb specimens of bud, close-ups of crystallized nugs, and carefully crafted joints. Internet users are now looking for a different kind of "weed porn." For example, Pornhub is reporting that searches for cannabis-related terms were 206% higher than average on Legalization Day in Canada. According to the porno website, searches that included terms such as "420", "smoking weed", "weed sex", "horny weed", "girls smoking weed", "ganja girls", and "smoking weed blowjob" topped the charts on October 17.

Search the hashtag #ganjagirls on Instagram and you will get more than a million hits featuring photo after photo of women posing provocatively with weed. Some of the models are promoting their own businesses and products like glassware or edibles, while others are just straight up getting high—and attempting to look seductive while they are at it.

Porn sites like Pornhub and YouPorn now boast thousands of amateur and professional smutty videos starring cannabis use.

Countless porn-star-produced clips, custom videos, and cam shows across the Internet showcase performers partaking in an ever-more-legal pastime. As cannabis becomes increasingly legal, it is finding its way into porn. Both of the two taboos carries its own stigma, misinformation from the outside, even though both are multi-billion-dollar industries. Many people with weed fetishes, are literally turned on by seeing the way that the light that reflects off the smoke, and the hazy diffusion that smoke leaves behind. Add beautiful women to the mix and you have a very visually appealing product. Smoking can be sexy, whether you are a fetishist or not. After all, you are watching a phallic-looking thing go into a mouth, watching it getting sucked on and watching white stuff come out. For smoking fetishists, weed porn can scratch several quite particular itches. Ela Darling, a cam performer, TEDx speaker and VR content manager of CAM4VR, has filmed quite a bit of smoking porn herself, and claims it is the minutiae to which masturbating viewers pay so much attention. Whether performers keep their fingers on the cigarette, or let it go when they take a drag. The way the mouth moves, even the way they exhale. Those details have long centred around cigarettes, but they can easily translate to smoking a joint too.

Kendra Sunderland, retired porn star does very well, thank you very much from weed related merchandise, including her own brand of rolling papers and grinders and lighters. Weed merchandising is becoming more accessible as the industry becomes more legal, and some porn stars have even gone so far as to brand their own strains of weed, like now-retired Skin Diamond. Some performers even claim that sharing their smoking habit with fans is a great way to be more relatable.

Building on their well-known brand recognition, "alt-pin-up-girl" Tumblr-style blog site, Suicide Girls recently launched a cannabis brand. Their product line is built on three distinct vape cartridges focusing specifically on the effects most beloved by their models—Chill, Hustle, and Zero. Chill is an anti anxiety strain, while Hustle is very much the opposite. Zero boasts anti-munchie effects, thanks to the presence of THCV, a cannabinoid that has been found to suppress appetite and regulate blood sugar, and is one of the few cannabis products that does leave you wanting to devour the refrigerator. The sleek metal vape pens demonstrate how thoughtful design is becoming a priority in the cannabis space, and at 65% THC per pen, they pack a pretty powerful hit. They also shows the huge potential profits that are available in this burgeoning marketplace, retailing at $55 for a one-gram cartridge.

On traditional porn sets, most companies require performers to verify that they are not under the influence of any alcohol or drugs. Ironically, even at Emerald Triangle Girls, who specialize in lesbian stoner porn, the weed the performers smoke on camera is fake. But not every set is so strict about intoxication. After all, cannabis is frequently prescribed as a medicine, and few directors prohibit their talent from medicating themselves. For porn performers, whose jobs require them to be relaxed, present, and very much aware of their bodies, cannabis is almost a foregone conclusion. Most webcam platforms discourage the use of intoxicants, but there are so many people camming at any given time that the odds of being caught are virtually non-existent.

Canna-Erotica

Although XXX platforms prohibit cannabis use on camera, cam girls have also noticed the benefits of adopting a stoner-girl persona. Searching for "420" and other cannabis keywords returns a huge numbers of hits, including perennial page 1s and even top-row models. Large numbers of Manyvids models appear to have built their brand around marijuana use, using drug-related terms in their names and profiles. Streamate, MyFreeCams, Chaturbate and iWantClips all feature models offering bong hits and much, much more for tips. A search for weed of Clips4Sale returned unexpected results, as apparently, watching hot women weed the garden is a growing niche fetish. Despite this, you can also find thousands of videos clearly depicting cannabis use. Although drug use is a clear agreement violation, FanCentro (part of the ModelCentro organization) ran a "420" promotional contest for their models, encouraging explicit depictions of the use of weed, so that is probably a good measure of how seriously these sites enforce their own policies.

Weed Girls and The Ganja Girls are both relatively new sites that feature hot models exploring the more sensual side of marijuana. Taking this one stage further, Emerald Triangle Girls is a women-owned adult production company formed in 2015, that specializes in lesbian stoner porn and who now put out a new DVD of material about every six weeks. They do a lot of unique on-camera interviews; they interview the girls about their usage, how they started, that sort of thing, so there is a little bit of that reality aspect, but instead of it having a reality look, it comes across more like a 20/20 interview. They combine beautiful erotic scenes with marijuana, resulting in a product that seems more high-end, rather than the usual 'let's get stoned' party attitude. Some of the most popular titles include the Hot Box, Girl Kush and Girl Kush 2 featuring stoner, biker chicks and blazing hot lesbian sex.

Despite the lesbian focus, Emerald videos, like most weed porn, are aimed squarely at the male audience. At the moment, there is unfortunately not a great deal of cannabis-related erotica for women available. In my experience, we females tend to prefer carefully crafted words, rather than the hardcore close-ups that are so popular in video porn. Even so, there remains a distinct dearth of literary offerings in this new sub-genre. I hope that this book might inspire you to fill this gap. If you would like to take a peek at my own efforts, 'Late Night at the Dispensary' is listed in the final chapter of this book, entitled 'More Titles from the Borderland Press.' In addition to my own first foray, one of the publisher's most prolific authors also has an offering entitled 'Tantric Tales of Tibetan Lust.' Please bear in mind that all authors in the Borderlands stable receive a cash bonus whenever you leave us a review on Amazon, so thank you in advance, on behalf of us all.

Cannabis Tourism

If you are not lucky enough to have wild cannabis plants growing on the other side of your back-yard fence, a quick search of the internet will reveal a cannabis connoisseur's atlas of Asia, with many places of pilgrimage for ganja gourmets. Varanassi in India, Baguio in the Philippines, Dali in China and Siem Reap in Cambodia are all perennially popular destinations for cannabis fans. Lijiang is well-known as the holiday romance capital of China, and many singles make the journey up into the foothills in the hope of finding a holiday hook-up. The most popular attraction in the area is a hike along the famous Tiger Leaping Gorge, which is twice as deep as the Grand Canyon, and where cannabis grows wild at every turn. Unfortunately, cannabis is still highly illegal in China and so there is still quite some risk involved.

In the meantime, it is still possible to organise a 'Himalayan Cannabis Tour' on the other side of the plateau, with the Nepal based tour operator Upper Himalayan Treks and Adventure. For just $499.00, the tour combines the natural beauty of the Himalayan mountains, the rich cultural heritage of Nepal, and more wild growing cannabis than you have ever seen in your life. Highlights include visits to historic and culturally significant areas that relate directly to Cannabis such as Freak Street and Pashupatinath temple as well as tours of farms in rural areas of Nepal to see their horticultural practices. Continuous mountain vistas that will take your breath away are obviously a given in these locations. For more details please email 'upperhimalaynadventures@gmail.com.'

While you might not be able to make it up to the majestic peaks surrounding Mopu Palace, there are a selection of self-appointed gurus out there hosting tantric THC retreats. An interesting example is the Pleasure Peaks Tantric Cannabis Couples Retreat which took place at a Muskoka mansion in Ontario, was described a heady trifecta of sex, spirituality and cannabis designed to encourage new levels of intimacy, trust and pleasure. Tantric sex instructor Antuanette Gomez, focuses on practical exercises to bring couples closer. Each day, an optional three-hour tantra workshop explores energy balance, erotic massage techniques, and even genital work using easy-to-understand diagrams. There is unfortunately, a policy of no public nudity and so anybody anticipating a full-blown Bacchanalian orgy will, for the time being, have to look elsewhere. Instead, her events include all meals, and cannabis-infused aphrodisiacs with each course. Couples receive customized vape pens, flower, and access to a dab bar. CBD pens are also on hand to help ground any guests who feel too high. As well as cannabis-infused gastronomy and tantric sexercise, the luxurious mansion includes a heated indoor pool, hot tub, and sauna and tickets are $1795 per couple.

Cannabis tourism is now growing rapidly throughout North America. The Colorado Department of Revenue said the state attracted some 6.5 million cannabis tourists in 2016, a number that is growing by around 10% per annum.

Colorado is pioneering this movement with luxury digs like Nativ Hotel downtown, where half the rooms come with balconies where smoking and vaping is allowed, and the B&B Adagio, which offers six historic suites designed specifically with the cannabis connoisseur in mind. The Marijuana Business Factbook estimates the economic impact of legal marijuana will increase 223% from 2017 to 2022. Colorado found that the more touristy the area of the state, the more marijuana costs, which in turn generates higher sales tax revenues. Last year, cannabis sales outpaced alcohol sales in Aspen for the first time. Additionally, towns near the border with states where cannabis use is not legalized have significantly higher per capita sales than interior areas. That out-of-state market of potential day-trippers is just waiting to be tapped. Colorado, Native Roots, a dispensary chain with 20 locations that claims to be the world's largest, says that about 36 percent of its customers come from out of state. Clearly, travellers are interested in marijuana. A Denver-based company called City Sessions offers tours targeting everybody from those interested in getting into the cannabis business themselves to beginners visiting from elsewhere, like the Mile High Sightseeing trip, which starts with a tour of a commercial grow facility and a visit to a dispensary, followed by a scenic drive through the city or up to the famed Red Rocks Amphitheatre. City Sessions also offers a New to Cannabis tour with a full introduction to cannabis production and consumption (even including a glass-blowing demo). Last year, City Sessions ran 288 tours ranging in size from a single person to groups of 50, seeing just over 1,000 customers in total. The owners have been astounded by the diversity of customers. "Last week, we had a group of five women all between 63 and 72 years old in from Iowa. It's really hard to bucket them in terms of age or gender, whether they're new to cannabis or a connoisseur."

In 2015, Oregon became the third state to legalize recreational marijuana. In Portland, the Jupiter Hotel has partnered with local cannabis businesses to create the 420 Package, which includes an issue of Oregon Leaf magazine, a vape pen and a package of coupons and other goodies from nearby dispensaries. It quickly became their best-selling package ever, opening up a whole new market segment. For now, state and local tourism-promotion organizations have stayed mostly silent on cannabis and tourism, but there are hints of change there, too. Even the mayor realises that cannabis as an industry not unlike other industries that have made Portland famous, such as craft breweries and craft distilleries. That said, Travel Portland's current policy is that it will not fund any cannabis-related activities or accompany media members to dispensaries.

Travel Portland is receiving so many inquiries from journalists they predict that they will soon be talking about recreational cannabis and strains that are only available in Portland in the same way we do about farm-to-table cuisine. Ads urging visitors to come use marijuana in Portland are certainly not far off. For the moment, even guests at the Jupiter Hotel who take advantage of the 420 Package are not technically allowed to enjoy any cannabis in their rooms. To get around this, they are supplied with odourless, smokeless vape pen, on the basis that what people do in the privacy of their own room is their own business. If the management cannot smell it or see it, then they do not know it has happened.

Meanwhile, in California, "wine and weed" tours are becoming increasingly more popular. Party buses, with the driver sealed off from smoking passengers, tour wineries and dispensaries, allowing tourists to sample the various products on offer. Across the country there are also "puff and paint" events, featuring cannabis tastings, wine and the chance to paint your own masterpiece. One tour company plays on the mystique of cannabis, offering tours "behind the curtain" of the legal marijuana industry in six states, along with some sampling along the way. Major newspapers such as the San Francisco Chronicle now feature travel-section stories detailing the "five best places for marijuana tourism," highlighting luxury cannabis getaways and DIY holidays.

Marijuana tour companies are becoming some of the first to truly embrace pot tourism with truly innovative experiences such as an introspective stroll through the ancient Redwood Forest of Humboldt County, under the semi-psychedelic influence of a Jack Flash infused brownie. Emerald Farm Tours in Northern California offers a San Francisco cannabis culture and city tour as well as an outdoor marijuana farm tour in Sonoma County which sell out consistently. The Ganja Goddess Getaway, is a San Francisco wellness retreat designed for women who already love cannabis, as well as those who want a safe space to try it for the first time. The schedule includes a weekend of yoga, educational classes, spa treatments — and unlimited cannabis in every form imaginable, including smoothies, body creams and vapes. The co-founder Deidra Bagdasarian, who also created Bliss Edibles, now one of the premier cannabis confectioneries in the U.S. has had so much interest in her "glamp-out" cannabis weekends that she is now expanding across the country and overseas.

In Canada, Butiq Escapes is a luxury weed tourism company based out of Victoria, British Columbia, They offer hiking in the spectacular Cascade Range for $12,500, where a guide picks you up from a private airport, smokes with you in the mountains and feeds you (and up to a group of four), lunch and dinner. With Canadians slated to spend $7 billion on marijuana sales in 2019, it is really no surprise there is a new wave of luxury weed tourism companies popping up. They offer bespoke itineraries for high-end tourists who want weed in style. Since October 17, Canadian Kush Tours in Toronto have hosted over a dozen private tours, from a smoked-out tours of upscale vapour lounges to a cannabis wedding bar for $3,000. Canna Tours, in Victoria, BC, has also seen a surge in bookings, as they tend to draw the VIP bachelor party crowd offering VIP access at local nightclubs. They also offer custom packages to cannabis events like 420 celebrations in Vancouver and music festivals which are very popular and sell out quickly. Other customers seem to enjoy learning about the different kinds of ways to consume cannabis and how the different benefits of how topical, edibles, and concentrated cannabis can be an alternative to the traditional method of just smoking the plant. The Ste. Anne's Spa in Grafton, Ontario, offers cannabis massage treatments with hemp CBD oil, for $155. People are going to be coming to Canada looking for legal weed, looking for places to consume and hotels that are cannabis-friendly such as the Bud and Breakfast Teapot House in BC. Bud and Breakfast for an Airbnb-style selection of international rooms and properties, including everything from cabanas on the white sand beaches of Ibiza, Spain, to lodges in the temperate rainforests of Homer, Alaska. Every listing is completely cannabis friendly and many come furnished with bongs, vaporizer rigs, or infused welcome mints, so you don't even have to travel with your paraphernalia.

Nevada, perhaps unsurprisingly as the home of Sin City, is ahead of the curve on cannabis tourism, despite the fact that cannabis use is outlawed on the Vegas Strip. Marijuana revenue last year exceeded expectations by 25%, generating new tax revenue of around $70 million for the state but with only four places in America—Idaho, South Dakota, Nebraska and Kansas—which still ban marijuana entirely, domestic cannabis tourism may not last much longer, especially if there is federal legalisation in 2020.

According to research in Amsterdam, 25 to 30 per cent of tourists come for a Dutch cannabis coffee shop experience. While coffee shops across the Netherlands have been satisfying visitors' weed needs for 50 years, cannabis is now decriminalised for recreational purposes, at least in part, in nearly 40 countries. It can now be legally consumed in five countries (although Georgia and South Africa allow possession and consumption but outlaw sales). In places where cannabis remains illegal, like England for example, organizations like the London Cannabis Club hold meet ups and events, including smoke-outs in public locations and private dinner parties where marijuana is cooked right into the main dish. Organizations like this are also intensely active in the fight to legalize cannabis locally, and can both inform and connect you before you arrive in "The Big Smoke." Even in countries that do not persecute cannabis, like Spain, Barcelona is earning a reputation as the "New Amsterdam" due to the proliferation of cannabis clubs. Connecting before arriving is clearly an intelligent move. Almost all of Barcelona's 350-plus cannabis clubs are members only, meaning you cannot simply show up and join the party unannounced. However, Cannabis Barcelona can set you up before your trip with everything you are going to need when you arrive.

At the moment, the legal-cannabis business is kind of the Wild West, with a patchwork of unclear regulations that vary from state to state, and even city to city. Advertising on Google and social media outlets like Facebook are hugely important for hotels and many other tourist-focused businesses, but the companies severely restrict what cannabis businesses are allowed to do.

Nothing beats the experience of a romantic getaway, so if you own government is still in the dark ages regarding drug legislation, please consider some of these innovative options. If we can show the opposition that we are willing to spend money to go to places that have enlightened drug policies, they will have little choice but make appropriate changes.

Modern Cannaphrodisiacs

A range of new start-ups are just starting to take advantage of the aphrodisiac qualities of cannabis and are releasing an exciting range of breakthrough products that can be incorporated into the bedroom. New in the west anyway. Some of the most innovative and revolutionary products for women's health are coming out of the cannabis industry. Such products include: PMS-relieving suppositories, bath salts, and tinctures; female-specific sexual-enhancement lubes; libido-boosting teas, chocolates, and vape pens; and more. Some even combine the aphrodisiac properties with improved vaginal health and wellness. I am sure that it will not be long before we see the modern equivalent of cann-aphrodisiac Tupperware parties, maybe even the return of Passion Parties and Ann Summers' sex toy parties with a distinct cannabis twist. At least I hope so.

Unfortunately, many of these products have severely limited availability at the moment. Some are only available in liberally-leaning California while others will require a visit to Colorado or even Alaska. You will even need to trek deep into the Tibetan Borderlands to sample The Princess Whisperer.

Somewhat surprisingly, the vast majority of cannaphrodisiacs are aimed at the ladies. I say surprisingly because traditional aphrodisiacs have long been the domain of horny, older guys. If only these products were available in China, perhaps we could bring tigers and rhinos back from the brink of extinction. The other thing is that many of these products are clearly masturbatory aids, and again this has long been a practice dominated by teenage boys and the dirty mac brigade. In some ways, it seems unfair that the act of jacking off is so horribly maligned for men, and yet becoming so widely acceptable for women. Men that are reduced to latex lovers are seen as losers of the worst kind, while women who enjoy dildos and vibrators are seen as forward thinking feminists.

Perhaps this is because so many women have problems achieving orgasm while horny males seem to be able to knock them out with little more than a few furtive strokes of the hand. If some of this stigma could be overcome, then I am sure that there would be a huge market for cann-aphrodisiacs squarely aimed at male consumers. It is as not as if there would be any shortage of willing beta-testers. I am sure that there would be a queue of randy young men queuing up around the block to try out the latest strains bred specifically to enhance male stimulation.

Many of the cannabis sex enhancement oils are actually aimed at women suffering from menstrual cramps. Actually, people have been using marijuana to deal with menstrual pain for a very long time — Queen Victoria was even said to employ the help of cannabis for just this purpose. These compounds have proven to be remarkably safe for human consumption for over 10,000 years. Now, with legalization taking America by storm, more and more women are finding the relief they need from painful menstrual cramps, usually after they have tried everything else — prescription pain medication, traditional Chinese herbs, acupuncture, massage, even witchcraft.

Always start with applying to a small area first to check for any adverse reactions. A good area to test is on your inner arm before applying to vaginal tissue. Check for swelling, redness, itching or burning. It can take up to 24 hours to react. Do not use any further if you experience an adverse reaction.

Dosage is another knob you can fiddle with, in order to dial in on the perfect level. 2.5mg is a good place to start as a beginner. Tinctures are the easiest for micro dosing. For anyone who is prone to anxiety (which THC can cause or exacerbate at higher doses)—this can make it very difficult to experience pleasure. Once you find the dosage that it best for you, you might even find that your period can actually be enjoyable.

Be aware that prescription depression medications can have a negative effect on masturbation and orgasming. They can even lead to loss of sex drive or orgasm (sometimes called anorgasmia). Anti-anxiety meds maintain higher levels of serotonin—which is what SSRIs and SNRIs such as Effexor both do, keeping serotonin around in the brain and nervous system longer, boosting emotional regulation—sexual drive is decreased. These medications also have an impact on dopamine and oxytocin as well, two neurotransmitters vital in emotional experiences such as falling in love, maternal bonding, and sexual pleasure or desire. In addition, undergoing any kind of life stress, whether it is financial difficulty, problems with a partner, family drama, unhappiness at work, or even mental illness can all have similar effects.

Foria are true innovators in female-specific CBD products, and the market leader when it comes to developing cannabis for menstrual relief and sexual enhancement, and women everywhere are grateful. The company champions sustainability and pride themselves on being organic. They are one of the few companies to use 100% organic MCT oil made exclusively from coconuts rather than environmentally destructive palm oil. The Colorado growing operation that they source from received the Conservationist of the Year Award from the National Resources Conservation Service due to their dedication to soil and water enhancement.

Foria is best known for its original product, Foria Relief: a cannabis vaginal suppository that specifically targets menstrual pain. To say it was well-received is an understatement. This all-natural solution to period pain has been featured in the New York Times, Cosmopolitan, and GQ, just to name a few. Patients with conditions like vaginismus, PCOS or vulvodynia have reported similar, non-menstrual-cycle-related experiences. For many women, the only previous resource were opiates that simply shut off the pain receptors, so that all feeling was eliminated. Although they are often called "weed tampons," Foria suppositories are not meant to absorb menstrual blood, but they do block pain receptors in the uterus. Endometriosis sufferers can use them in a non-sexual manner during an endo flare, and they can even be used as a massage oil. Foria lubes are not condom compatible. In fact no oil based lubes are going to be compatible with condoms.

Foria has since expanded its product line to include non-THC offerings (Foria Relief and their other THC-laden products are only available in California and Colorado) that enhance the natural benefits of CBD by adding organic botanicals and essential oils. Some customers describe the therapeutic effects as a complete vaginal melt down, feeling like it emulsified every tense muscle in the lower body.

"It was like all my pelvis muscles had been holding their breath and suddenly let it out, all at once. It was magic. I may have cried. It was like mainlining medicine straight to my uterus muscles."

Many users experienced incredible relief and slept better than ever.

Prior to administering Foria relief, one reviewer complained of constant disruption from excruciating pain in her internal organs and debilitating cramps, She felt as though her inflamed uterus had expanded to fill her entire midsection, leaving her feeling bloated, nauseous, and feeling as though she was auditioning for the role of John Hurt's understudy in Alien.

It is a good idea to pop the suppository into the freezer for 15 minutes to make sure that the small, white, pearl-sized bullet is firm. They are slippery little devils and you do not want them dissolving in your hand. Launch the tiny torpedo straight into your honey pot and it will be on a fast track directly to your cervix. There is an ahhhhh-mazing creamy, buttery chocolate and coconut scent and warm, golden waves will soon be emanating from my vagina throughout the rest of my body. All of the muscles that had been cramped and clenched so tight gradual released and your body can relax again.

"Where I had been painfully aware of every inch of my midsection, suddenly it felt as though I had no midsection at all. From my waist down to my thighs, it was almost as if my groin had simply dissolved and was floating in some galaxy far, far away."

At $44 for four suppositories, Foria is not cheap. They are best for use before bed — or at least when you are not about to stand up right after (because you want the medicine to stay up in there and not drip out). It is a good idea to wear some panties with a liner which will help catch oil that might leak out if you get up too soon after inserting. Alternatively, sit back for 15-20 minutes and relax a little. While the relief is palpable and pronounced, it is unfortunately short-lived. It takes about 20 minutes before you begin to feel the effects, which, last for about an hour. But what a glorious hour it is. Each serving has 60mg of THC and 10mg of CBD, but it will not make you feel high — it just alleviates all your pain. Here's to a future world where everyone with cramps can access these pain management materials without fear of the law.

Foria lube comes in two types - Foria Pleasure, which is the one that has THC, and Foria Awaken, which is their THC-free line made with CBD and kava. Foria Pleasure is an 1 oz bottle with 2.5mg of THC per spray that also retails for $44. The spray is made of cannabis oil and coconut oil, not only keeping everything nice and slick down there, but also enhancing sensation all over. It is actually a pre-lube that requires 25 minutes for the THC to absorb into the mucosal membranes. The company says that Foria Pleasure "brings the power of ancient plant medicine to your fingertips." Named the "Sex Product of the Year" by GQ in 2014 when it first hit the shelves, Foria Pleasure claims that "for some women, it can help promote natural lubrication, reduce pain and tension and create the relaxation necessary for sensual experience or restorative rest."

For the rest of us, Foria Pleasure transforms us into lustful little pleasure monsters. It heightens all of your senses, increases your libido, and will change the way you orgasm. It does not necessarily bring you to orgasm faster (although for some, it can, since it can increase arousal), but it is the grand finale where you really feel major the results. Climaxes are deeper, all-consuming and way more intense than anything you have ever experienced before. Best of all, it will not make your vagina smell and taste like dirty old bong water. Your partner will not notice any distracting tastes or smells, nor will you or your vagina will see any swirly colours or talking lampshades, because the THC is not absorbed into the bloodstream when applied to the vagina. However, if you ingest the lube orally or use it anally, there is a chance of getting high, depending on your tolerance.

Sex blogger Liz Klinger used her Lioness vibrator to track

arousal and orgasm by measuring how her pelvic floor muscles and vaginal walls were squeezing during the masturbation session.

"Holy Krakatoa! With the Foria lube, not only did the orgasm itself feel deeper and more intense, it was like that for the entire masturbation session. My whole body felt more relaxed, open, and naturally lubricated than normal. I felt an increase in arousal, allowing me to be fully immersed in the enjoyment. I read a review on Foria's website that described it as "stimulation in HD," which is basically the best way to describe the sensation. My orgasm was 9x longer than normal. My orgasms normally are about 10-20 seconds long, but with the Foria lube, my orgasm lasted about 3 whole minutes. My orgasm was way more intense. My normal sessions don't have very much range in my vaginal wall muscles squeezing and relaxing before the orgasm. However, with the Foria lube, my vaginal muscles were squeezing and relaxing like crazy due to the heightened sensitivity and arousal, giving me an overall stronger orgasm."

Foria Explore is a cannabis suppository that is available in California and Colorado only, but promoted as "sensual enhancement and comfort during anal play." Explore delivers 60 mg of THC and 10 mg of CBD to "so you can experience muscle-relaxation and enhanced pleasure without the strong psychoactive effect traditionally associated with cannabis."

Foria Awaken is "full-spectrum hemp oil" with eight plant-based aphrodisiacs and a chocolate and mint aroma, that promotes relaxation through its synergistic combination of CBD, kava root, organic cardamom, and other potent ingredients. It comes in a spray bottle and the dominating smell is a soft mint – similar to the smell of mint chocolate chip ice cream, so be prepared for your lover to nickname you the peppermint pussy!

The spray application makes it very easy and clean to use. No more soaking heavy silicone based lubricants on your sheets or staining your clothes.

Their latest non-THC product, Foria Flow, is a high-quality vape pen that delivers CBD with a blend of terpenes and essential oils for a smooth experience. It is reusable, unlike many CBD vape pens and is yet another example of Foria's eco-conscious practices. They cost $88 for 30 ml (approximately 30 "servings") or $24 for 5 ml (about five servings).

Whoopi and Maya

After suffering from severe menstrual cramps and then watching her daughter and granddaughters go through the same agony, Whoopi Goldberg partnered with Om Edibles founder Maya Elisabeth launched a line of products to spare women everywhere this agonising experience. I was a little skeptical about a celebrity sponsored line of products, especially when I learned that they employed a "head herbalist/wizard-in-residence," but the salve, tincture, bath soak, and edible chocolates all provide luxurious cures for extreme period pains. There are also two tinctures available – THC only and CBD heavy. The Whoopi & Maya "Relax" THC Herbal Tincture has approximately 50 mg THC in a 2 oz jar and approximately 100 mg THC in a 4 oz jar. A 1 oz bottle costs $27-30 and a 2oz one for $45-50. The CBD-heavy botanical formula has 40 mg CBD and approximately 2 mg THC in a 2 oz jar and 80 mg CBD and approximately 4 mg THC in an 8 oz jar. If you need quick relief from endometriosis, dysmenorrhea and PMS or severely painful periods that last several hours, this potent tincture can deliver. With a 15:1 ratio of CBD to THC, this works like magic in just five minutes. Not only does it erase the pain, but it does not leave anything else in its place, leaving you feeling fully functional and normal. It is olive oil-based and therefore not the most delicious taste, but you can wash it down easily with pretty much anything you like. It is one of the most expensive products on the market at $60 a ml, most likely because CBD is a lot harder to extract than just making a tincture with cannabis as-is, which is mostly THC.

Whoopi & Maya "Soak" Bath Salts combine Epsom salts with cannabis, apricot kernel oil, avocado seed oil, jojoba oil, vitamin E, aloe vera, and essential oils. A 30-minute soak induces increasingly relaxed and bendy feelings with cramps being relieved after just a few minutes, which lasts for around five or six hours. This is a THC-heavy product — 25mg of THC per 8 oz container, retailing for $12-$15, but due to the strength, you only need to start off with a third of a jar. The salts make the bottom of the bathtub a bit slick, so beware of slips, and if you share the bathroom, make sure you scrub down the tub after so you do not accidentally dose whichever room-mate decides to bathe next.

A 2 oz tub of Whoopi & Maya "Savor" THC Raw Cacao retails for $14 to $18, with a 4 oz tub going for $27 to $30 and can be used to make hot chocolate, poured over ice cream, or just eaten by the spoonful. Although it was made for massage, the Whoopi & Maya "Rub" Body Balm is great for making DIY suppositories. Simply freeze little scoops into tiny balls, although scooping some of the balm directly into your vagina works just as well if you do not like that icy sensation. For both of these, expect a little numbness, but not anything scary or annoying. It retails at $20 for a 2 oz tin and $40 for a 4 oz tin.

Dr. Kerklaan Therapeutics Natural PMS Cream was designed by Andrew Kerklaan, a holistically-minded Canadian chiropractor who turned to cannabis topicals after more than 20 years of experience trying to manage his patients' pain. It uses a proprietary formulation, designed specifically to treat physical symptoms of PMS such as cramping.

A line of CBD-based lubricants called Privy Peach is meant to quell inflammation and increase circulation, which may in turn improve sexual function and arousal in women with problems such as endometriosis and other types of chronic pelvic pain.

Quim Rock Intimate Oil is a hand-made by Cyo Ray Nystrom and Rachel Washtein in San Francisco. They make topicals strictly designed for female pleasure, using the slogan, "Self-care for humans with vaginas." It comes in a Curious formula and a Sensitive formula, which are both specifically designed to intensify climax, enhance sensation, increase libido, and serve as a vaginal health supplement. Curious contains a small amount of tea tree oil, which is added for its antiseptic qualities, and they recommend 6-8 pumps or 8-10 mg THC and applying 20 minutes before sex. A 2 oz bottle with 193mg of THC retails for $46.

The Ancient Medicinal Herbs Company produces a number of Vajikarana Formulas, with the flagship product being called the God & Goddess Vitality Blends. Ayurvedic Wisdom states that there are 3 Pillars that uphold Vital Health and Longevity, which are:

1. Harmonious Diet- Supplemented with Rasayanas (Deeply Nourishing Tonic Herbal Formulas)

2. Harmonious Sleep cycles and Meditation practices

3. Harmonious Sexual Energy and its Wise Management

The Vajikarana Formulas include a number of ingredients as well as CBDs that are traditionally included in Ayurevedic and Chinese medicine. These include Shatavari (wild asparagus root), goji berries, schizandra berries, dong quai, Ashwagandha, damiana, tribulus, tulsi (holy basil), Fo Ti, cinnamon bark. While the efficacy of the additional ingredients, may not be as obvious as that of the cannabis plant, it is good to know that these artisans are incorporating items that have been used for thousands of years in folk medicine.

Described as being authentic Vajikaranas, these blends will enhance sex drive and help build Ojas, which is the source of a robust immunity, endurance, inner contentment.

HerbaBuena Quiver Sensual Cannabis Lubricant is a "sensual lubricant that increases pleasure, heightens sensitivity and supports and extend female orgasm." but also "tones soft tissue, eases painful intercourse and alleviates menstrual cramps." Quiver was voted Best Sensual Product by SF Chronicle Green State in 2017. A 2-ounce bottle contains 84mg of THC blended with cinnamon and cloves in an organic coconut oil base. The producers recommend two pumps to start with, equalling about 4mg of THC.

Humboldt Apothecary sells both a "Cramp Ease" product, and a sex enhancer which is very appropriately called "Love Potion #7." The PMS product is a mild tincture to be taken under the tongue, which utilizes a 1:1 ratio of THC to CBD. It also includes cramp bark, which, as its name suggests, is used as a holistic treatment for cramps. This sex-centric Love Potion #7 can also be used as personal lubricant. It is a blend of natural, ethical ingredients, which include coconut MCT oil, damiana, cinnamon, kava kava, cardamom, roasted cocoa nibs, vanilla bean, vitamin E, stevia and 250 mg of THC.

Apothecanna Sexy Time Personal Intimacy Oil is an industrial hemp-derived CBD product, which can be purchased in all 50 states. The plant-based glide combines jasmine, argan, cannabis and coconut. Apothecanna's modest marketing explains that you can massage this oil onto "your neck, chest, and other erogenous zones" fifteen minutes before getting intimate.

Many chronic pain sufferers report the positive impacts that cannabis has on their sex lives. Even something as simple as a pulled muscle can make intimacy painfully uncomfortable and put a damper on your sex life. For these instances Apothecanna manufactures a 1:1 CBD:THC Extra Strength Pain Relieving Cream which works wonders on sports injuries.

Stoney Yoni comes in two variations: Stoney Yoni and Stoney Yoni Essential Health. The former is a "personal massage oil" with 160mg of THC per bottle to stimulate lubrication and promote sensitivity. The Essential Health version is more "therapeutic" with anti-fungal, anti-bacterial and anti-inflammatory properties and also contains rose, lavender and chamomile.

Luminous Botanicals DEW also comes in two versions. When applied as a sensual lubricant, the original high THC blend enhances sensitivity, while the Balanced THC/CBD blend reduces discomfort. DEW is made with all organic, food-grade ingredients, including Clean Green Certified cannabis.

Bare Spray is a personal lubricant made with organic, fractionated coconut oil, essential oils, and cannabis oil concentrate derived using CO_2 extraction "with flower containing zero chemical pesticides and no hydrocarbons." Safe to ingest – the formula was approved by the state's marijuana control board as an edible. Five pumps equals 5mg of THC and the essential oils include bergamot, ylang ylang, lavender, clary sage, rose, cinnamon leaf, sweet orange, sandalwood, neroli and jasmine.

Velvet Swing was founded by Mistress Matisse when she realized the power of cannabis to enhance people's sex lives. It is also worth noting Velvet Swing is water-based/water-soluble and safe for latex condom use. It is a 0.44 oz bottle with 1.5mg of THC and 0.5mg of CBD per spray and retails for $49. Velvet Swing offers partners of all genders the opportunity of long, strong orgasms—with occasional tingling and coolness experienced by some fans.

"Love Your Ladyparts" Skin Balm retails for $32 for a 2.7 oz jar and is designed and marketed for use on skin, the vulva, and inside the vagina. Trying putting a heaped spoonful inside and letting it melt into your pussy walls. It might be a bit messy, but a spoonful of anything in there is going to create some mess as you cannot remain horizontal forever.

The fact that weed culture is still heavily male oriented has led to the launch of an all female cannabis delivery service called Lady Chatterley's Lover in California. The company employs a team of highly knowledgeable ladies as "product consultants," and is a wonderful alternative to calling up some dodgy dealer down in the ghetto.

I would also like to include here two of my own favourite products here, which will probably be very difficult for most readers to obtain, but were my own first experiences into the realm of cannaphrodisiacs. Both of these oils are hand-crafted by a western trekking guide, who I met in the Himalayan foothills, midway between Lijiang and Shangri-La. Unfortunately, cannabis is technically illegal in China, even though it grows everywhere and the locals regularly use it as a source of protein. Most tourists view the smoked weed with disdain, simply because they do not know how to harness its magical powers. This particular high-altitude strain has to be used sparingly and infrequently to obtain the full effect, and works best as a tool of inspiration for artists and intellectuals, rather than a group sacrament for twenty-first century hippies, bent on getting hammered as quickly as possible. Here in the mystical mountains of Tibet, it will probably come as no surprise that it works best as a tantric stimulant, opening up pleasure receptors and releasing inhibitions. This is not the wheelchair weed that you find so commonly on the West Coast, cannabis that will put you in coma after a couple of puffs. This is a super-cerebral smoke that will bring out your inner Salvador Dali and your underlying Immanuel Kant. The oil and the seeds are both relatively THC free, but do retain large amounts of CBDs making them very useful health foods, although finding hulled kernels is as yet unknown.

It is grown mainly for the nutritious seed and super healthy oil, but is much more rarely used as a recreational. Once you get out of the city limits, you will start to see huge plantations of the stuff growing all over the countryside. Even in the towns, you will occasionally see monster plants springing up on plots of wasteland over the summer months. The police have ruled that locals can still grow it, as long as it is at least one hundred metres away from any public road. The idea here is that what is out of sight is out of mind, but you simply cannot help stumbling across it if you spend enough time in the area. The ongoing trade war has recently strengthened long-standing anti-foreigner prejudices among the Chinese, and the singling out of westerners for testing is now common place. It also does not help that there are large numbers of uninvited Christian missionaries in the area, stirring up problems for all the properly registered expats. Despite this persistent persecution by the local authorities, there is a very active underground artisanal scene in the popular tourist towns of Dali, Shaxi and Lijiang.

I was lucky enough to try two different blends which were

both truly amazing. The first was labelled as 'The Tibetan Crown of Conciousness,' sold as a hair thickener and applied as a scalp rub, but with amazing psychotropic side effects. The second had a label decorated with images of the erotic murals from the Blue Room at Mopu Palace and was aptly named 'The Princess Whisperer.' Unsurprisingly, this was an erotic oil designed to enhance the user's love life in ways that would put shivers up the spines of the poor, stricken sisters in Black Narcissus. This was a cann-aphrodisiac extract elixir that was guaranteed to turn even the most pious nun into a raving nymphomaniac. It was the delicate shade of baby coconuts and was suitable for everything from cooking to sacred rituals.

While China continues to rewrite its history and cut itself off from the rest of the world, I am sad to say that it will be very difficult for the rest of you to sample these exquisitely hand-crafted products for yourselves, but I do hope that they inspire you to try artisanal alternatives from far more enlightened countries around the world. I hope that you might even have a try at making your own.

DIY cannabis oil

For those that have the urge to give it a whirl but do not have access to a dispensary. Large scale cannabis companies that produce sexually-focused topicals use CO2 extracted cannabis oil mixed, but this requires six-figure extraction equipment, which the average consumer cannot replicate at home. For the hobbyist, and especially those living in prohibition areas, a method that is both simple and pragmatic is preferred.

Decarboxylation is a crucial step in any cannabis product's potency and efficacy It facilitates and edible recipe, and the creation of capsules, tinctures, or any other medicinal or recreational cannabis products. For the technically minded, plant based cannabinoids including THC and CBD, are locked in an acidic form, not bio-available to your cannabinoid receptors. The acidic form of THC is THCA, which is molecularly identical to THC – except for an additional carboxyl group. This carboxyl group prevents THCA from binding to your cannabinoid receptors. Much like keys and locks, cannabinoids need to be the correct shape to fit in our receptors, and therefore have an effect. Decarboxylation makes the THCA available to the cannabinoid receptors throughout your endocannabinoid system including in your brain and nervous system.

This may sound complicated but the release process is actually very easy. I have included very detailed instructions below, but can assure you that my own initial experiments did not include half of this equipment, and the final product still turned out to be amazing. There is no need to add essential oils or other additives to your oil. With this two ingredient method, your oil is endlessly versatile. Be warned: oil based lubes are not compatible with latex condoms, so always consider your backup protection methods carefully.

Ingredients

8 oz virgin coconut oil

¼ oz of bud

Equipment

Two 4 oz Mason jars

Food scales

Grinder

Slow cooker with a "warm" setting

Unbleached cheese cloth

Large funnel

Smaller funnel

Tincture bottle with a 1 mL calibrated pipette

Yields: Approximately 6mg of THC per 1mL of oil

Some people like to grind up their cannabis using a food processor, but I prefer to use a hand grinder. The THC is activated through a standard decarboxylation method: Spreading the ground cannabis evenly on a cookie sheet and baking in a preheated 240 degree Fahrenheit oven to for one hour on the middle rack. Stir at 30 minutes. Once the cannabis is decarboxylated, divide evenly into each 4 oz mason jar. In even proportions, add the oil to each jar.

Make sure the lid of the Mason jar is as tight as possible.

Place the Mason jars in the slow cooker and cover with boiling water so that the jars are fully submerged. Set slow cooker to "warm" setting for 4-5 hours.

Every 60 minutes, using a jar clamp or heavy oven mitts, pull out the jars and give them a good shake. Be careful not to burn yourself as the glass and metal will both be hot. While the mason jar method is great for containing the smell, decarboxilating is highly fragrant. If you have nosy neighbours, try frying bacon or cooking something comparably fragrant at the same time to mask the scent.

After 4-5 hours, remove the jars from the water and place

them on a cloth until they are cool (do not put it on a cold/hard surface as the glass could crack). Line a funnel with 4 layers of cheesecloth and place over a large glass measuring cup, methodically squeezing out any plant matter that remains. If you see bits of weed floating in your oil, strain it again. Using a smaller funnel, pour the oil into a tincture bottle with a 1 mL graduated pipette. Unless you are using lab-tested pesticides, mould and other contaminants free flower, it is going to be very difficult to accurately calculate potency.

Other Interesting Products

Some edibles are great for micro dosing, like To Whom It May Chocolates or Nature Nurse's Cocoa Cannabinoids, both of which are available in California and come in 2.5mg doses—just make sure you are buying from a reputable company that actually batch tests the potency of its products. Dark chocolate is considered an aphrodisiac on its own, but Lulu's Botanicals Arouse Chocolates consists of 70% Cacao with a 1:1 ratio of 5MG THC : 5MG CBD. Additional ingredients include stimulating Yerba Mate and Kola Nut, and plant-based aphrodisiacs including Damiana, Catuaba, and Cistanche.

Lulu's was founded by Louise "Lulu" Sharpe, who began by making regular (read: non-cannabis-inclusive) chocolates but has long been a cannabis advocate. As such, her eventual expansion into edibles was perhaps inevitable. Each piece contains what's considered a micro-dose of 5 mg of THC along with raw cacao, coconut sugar, CBD oil, vanilla bean, and sea salt.

Serra is an elegant and high-end shop selling the kind of artisanal and hipster-friendly products Portland is known for. It has partnered with local chocolatier Woodblock to create a special series of edibles that have become a best-seller.

Woodblock has the same 'bean-to-bar' philosophy as the 'seed-to-weed' control expressed by Serra. The result meticulously crafted chocolate, with the level of detail that connoisseurs demand.

Dosist Arouse and Passion Pens are both vape pens that come pre-loaded with either 50 or 200 consistent, precise doses—each time you pull a puff, it buzzes to let you know you have had enough. Dosist has engineered the formulas to increase sensitivity and pleasure while at the same time relaxing the body and mind. Each dose is just 2.25 mg. The blend contains the terpenes linalool for relaxation and farnesene for arousal and contains a ratio of 10:1 THC-to-CBD.

Though Kikoko offers several formulas, one, Sensuali-Tea, is specifically designed to address libido. Gaining in popularity in the ingestibles/edibles category are cannabis and CBD teas. Kikoko offers a variety of cannabis-infused herbal teas, and their website claims their Sensuali-Tea can "intensify orgasms." Ingredients include hibiscus, rose petals, orange peel, lavender, cardamom, cloves, licorice root and most importantly, organically grown Kikogold Cannabis, coming in at 7mg THC per tea bag.

Since garlic and bacon condoms are things you can buy (though whether you actually want to is another question), Cannadom's cannabis-flavoured condoms were bound to pop up at some point. These boast a "realistic cannabis flavour and smell," plus some blatantly stoner-friendly packaging.

There is no actual cannabis in the Ganja Vibes Mary Jane vibrator, but the plant did inspire the shape—which serves a purpose, according to one reviewer, who wrote that "the ridges give an even better experience with the vibrations."

Peter Piper's Pecker Puffer is a glass pipe dildo that two birds with one stoner. I highly recommend washing it after each use, though, regardless of what you are using it for.

A Few Minor Downsides

Potency obviously affects the outcome when using cannabis to improve sex. At low to moderate levels, enthusiasts report increased ability to communicate with their partner, and increased physical awareness. Remember that although, it might take longer to get up the mountain, the view is much more epic once you get there.

Some users reported that when they were "very stoned" they tended to be introverted and closed. Others said that when they were very stoned, they lost the ability to communicate with their bodies and could not perform sexual activity because their awareness was higher than the concrete world. Remember that if you ingest too much, you are much more likely to fall asleep that experience out of this world orgasms.

A follow-on to this is that in many people's experience the intense creativity and vivid imaginations that is released through cannabis is paid for in our unconscious hours. I am definitely one of those people for whom smoking ensures that my sleep is completely devoid of dreams. As more and more work is done in the field of lucid dreaming, it could be argued, that we are using an artificial method to access a state of mind that is already available to us, but one that most of us do not have sufficient training to properly access.

If you get into the use of using cannabis for solo stimulation, there is always the risk that you quickly descend into repetitive cycle of self-satisfaction. You would not be the first rat race indentured servant that became addicted to solitary onanism, simply because it is easier to bring yourself to the shaking seizures of convulsive orgasm than it is to go out and find a willing partner. In some parts of the world it is very difficult to overcome the local brainwashing that vilifies sexual activity of any kind and educate a new lover in the erotic arts.

With edibles, dose control is more difficult than with smoking or vaping. Label recommendations cannot be trusted. And edibles may take an hour to produce their effects, so while waiting to get high, some people feel tempted to eat more than they can comfortably handle. In states with legal recreational cannabis, almost all emergency room admissions have involved edibles— people eating too much and later regretting it—suggesting a need for careful experimentation with dosage and timing. Some medicinal edibles aimed at serious sickness sufferers have incredibly high doses. A cannabis chocolate bar with a label that states that it contains a dosage equivalent to seventeen joints might well be ideal for a chronic multiple sclerosis sufferer but may well knock the rest of us out for days on end.

Although medical and recreational cannabis use is now legal in many US states, you may be putting yourself at risk if you live elsewhere. Testing for illicit drug use is a reality for many workers in the western countries. Drug testing is mandatory for federal employees in the US, and although it is not required in the private sector, more employers are implementing some kind of drug screening. It is also being used more and more by overseas enforcement agencies to target foreign recreational users. At the time of writing, the Chinese police are repeatedly raiding watering holes favoured by expats and doing lock-ins to test everybody on site. They usually use imported American tests as

Chinese versions are still unreliable. It is therefore important to know whether CBD oils will result in a positive drug test for THC or cannabis?

The SAMHSA (Substance Abuse and Mental Health Services Administration) guidelines have become a worldwide standard, and a routine urine drug screen for cannabis use consists of an immunoassay with antibodies that are made to detect it, and its main metabolite, 11-nor-delta9-caboxy-THC (THC-COOH), with a cut-off level 50 ng/mL for a positive reading. Most research suggests that for infrequent or 'non-daily' users of cannabis, a typical joint (containing about 40mg to 50mg of THC) would result in a positive THC metabolite screen for up to two days at this cut-off level, while regular users could remain positive for weeks. Fortunately, this has very little cross-reactivity to other cannabinoids, such as CBD (cannabidiol), CBG (cannabigerol), CBN (cannabinol) which is good news consumers of CBD oil.

Most CBD oil contain only 1/10th to 1/300th of the THC concentration found in cannabis. Individuals using unusually large doses of a cannabinoid-rich oil product (above 1000-2000 mg of hemp oil daily) could theoretically test positive but anybody requiring such mega-doses would probably be so debilitated by their illness that they would be unlikely to go out let alone to go out partying. Remember that the cannabis effect is determined by the personality, psychology, intent, environment, and culture of the user.

An Exciting Future

As of 2019, ten states, the District of Columbia, and the Northern Mariana Islands have legalized recreational use of cannabis, while 33 states, Guam, Puerto Rico, the U.S. Virgin Islands and D.C. have legalized medical use of the drug. In America at least, it looks like lots of US states will be legalizing cannabis this year and next. Once the number of states that have legalised becomes 35, there is then the opportunity to make a constitutional amendment that will legalise nationwide on a federal basis. This major change, unlike any in our lifetime, is at the vanguard of a coming revolution. Imagine buying a joint as easily as you can buy a six-pack of Corona. Imagine the rap-song product placements. Imagine the Super Bowl ads.

But let's not jump the gun. Federal law enforcement agencies receive huge funds yet to combat cannabis and the private prison systems make huge profits from keeping users locked up. Politicians are always loathe to upset their real constituents, the ones who make the biggest donations. As nationwide legalization becomes closer and closer, we can certainly expect pharmaceutical and agricultural giants try to throw a spanner in the works, or at least move in and drive small scale entrepreneurs out of business. The CBD industry alone is poised to be a $2 billion business by 2022, and corporations can literally smell the money.

Big Pharma and Big Ag have been responsible for much of the money behind the lobbying efforts to keep cannabis illegal, as they have been since the 1930s when they realized the threat cheaply grown cannabis posed and still poses to their chemical empires. Du Pont's egregious behaviour in this area is well documented, as is that of the Hearst newsprint empire which still rakes in more than $10 billion a year to this day. Hemp makes higher quality paper than wood pulp but Hearst already produced all the newsprint for the whole of the US from huge tracts of forest that he also owned, and he was not going to let any competition threaten his monopoly.

But now, as the economy has cratered and millions of Americans have found themselves forced to rethink their livelihoods, there's a growing feeling that the country can no longer afford its long-standing prohibition on cannabis — a sense, for the first time since the Seventies, that pot could soon be made fully legal. On the national level, a Harvard economist has estimated that legalizing pot could save the government $13 billion annually in prohibition costs (including cops and prisons) and raise many tens of $billions more in annual revenues if cannabis is taxed — a potent argument at a time when local municipalities are being forced to slash services and cut public-sector jobs.

From California to downtown Detroit, there is a green revolution sweeping across the nation, as cannabis shows itself to be a huge growth industry. Fanning out from the Emerald Triangle — an area in Northern California comprising the adjoining counties of Mendocino, Humboldt and Trinity, cannabis seeds that were smuggled in by hippies from Afghanistan now dwarfs any other sector of the state's agricultural economy.

This is a rapidly a growing economic boom period for cannabis. There is even a Las Vegas has cannabis trade show. MJBizCon is held at the Las Vegas Convention Centre for three days, showcasing vendors, seminars, conferences, and exhibits dedicated to squeezing ever more dollars out of cannabis plants.

Nevada collected more than $69.8 million in cannabis tax revenue during the first year of recreational sales after it legalized the drug in 2017.

As soon as visitors step out the door of McCarran International Airport, they are greeted by Taxis wrapped in a MedMen cannabis ads. Downtown, the world's largest cannabis dispensary, Planet 13 is designed like a 112,000 square feet Apple store. There is a 24-hour dispensary, which accounts for 15,000 square feet of the space, selling Planet 13-branded medical and recreational cannabis products, like capsules, vapes and more.

Touted as a destination dispensary, the place is clearly built to bring in tourists. The attached distillery offers interactive and visual experiences for visitors, like synchronized 3D projections on the lobby walls and walkways lit with sensory activated LED lights, so a trail of coloured lights follows guests as they walk.

There are 13, 15-foot LED lotus flowers that can be controlled by visitors as interactive art pieces and do laser graffiti by drawing with "spray cans" that shoot laser beams onto a wall.

Currently only 40,000 square feet of the total space is being used, and there are plans for a nightclub, a coffee shop, a tasting room for cannabis-infused beer and wine and a lounge for consuming cannabis on-site if that is legalized and space for food. According to Lyft, another mega dispensary, Reef is now one of the most visited places in Vegas by their passengers. Inside it is like an airport and apparently as busy, but with no security gates or machine gun-toting guards seen at a lot of California dispensaries. They specialise in celebrity strains, such as Shango, who are the exclusive grower of Tommy Chong's Choice buds. With the current trendiness of the Slow Food movement and the memorization's of everyone from artisanal butchers to "rock-star farmers," it is inevitable that some growers will become celebrities.

Whereas cheap, mass-produced weed from Mexico and South America once dominated the U.S. market, thanks to the so-called "green rush," about half of the cannabis sold is now high-quality domestic product. Partly, this has to do with the tightening of the border after 9/11, making it more and more difficult to smuggle large quantities of pot. Home-grown bud often comes from "small-scale operators who painstakingly tend greenhouses and indoor gardens to produce the more potent, and expensive, product that consumers now demand." (THC levels of Mexican weed, while improving, hover around seven percent, whereas high-end weed in Northern California can reach THC levels of 20 percent.) The advancement of high-performance four-channel LED technology in combination with vertical hydroponic farming, is now producing yields approaching 750 grams per square foot, compared to the industry average of 39. Let's just hope that not all cannabis is grown under computer controlled LEDs using an atomic clock timer, each bud being hand trimmed by bearded, transgender hipsters. There is a real risk that the whole thing could be ruined by a bunch of pinky-lifting poseurs just like coffee.

Cannabis CBD products are now being manufactured specifically for pets. Some companies are claiming that CBD dog and cat treats can help pet owners treat cancer, epilepsy, osteoporosis, joint pain, and anxiety. The Yunnan Baiyao Group, a Chinese pharmaceutical company based in Kunming for example, is developing Himalayan strains for veterinary use. Studies have shown that plants grown in very high altitudes, which get exposure to more UVA and UVB, tend to have higher THC concentrations. In greenhouses, using specially tweaked LED lighting, growers have already increased THC content by 30%.

Although, scientists have long been prohibited from investigating the myriad uses and varieties of each major strain of this healthful herb, companies and individuals in the states that have legalised are catching up quickly. The Stanley Brothers in Colorado are using industrial hemp CBD to make oils, capsules, creams, and balms — even CBD for dogs — and it is all available on-line to be shipped anywhere in the country. The company got the name "Charlotte's Web" for their most popular product not from the children's book, but rather from Charlotte Figi, a young girl with a rare, severe form of epilepsy called Dravet Syndrome. Charlotte used to suffer dozens of seizures a day, until she started taking CBD oil, and in her first week, went from having 300 seizures to none.

CBD is one of more than 100 chemical compounds found in the cannabis plant, which includes both cannabis and hemp strains. While CBD can be extracted from cannabis plants, the Stanley brothers' products come from "industrial" hemp, which contains less than 0.3 percent naturally-occurring THC. An estimated 50 percent of hemp plants in America are currently being grown for CBD extraction, according to the Associated Press. CBD oil is not the same as hemp oil comes directly from hemp seeds, which contain negligible amounts of CBD. The Charlotte's Web products come from the leaves and flowers of the hemp plant, but still contain less than 0.3% THC. It is marketed as a dietary supplement under federal law of the United States, being classified as "industrial hemp", which is legal in all 50 states, and does not induce the psychoactive "high" typically associated with recreational cannabis strains that are high in THC.

As Colorado has legalized both the medicinal and recreational use of cannabis, many parents have flocked there with their suffering children. In October 2014, the Stanley brothers had a waiting list of "more than 12,000 families, who the media have termed "cannabis refugees", forced to flee states where cannabis is off limits. Unexpected consequences like this have shown that legalization is one massive experiment on the human brain. Even though it will take years for us to begin to understand the full consequences, at least it cannot be as disastrous as the introduction of social media.

Today, countries all over the world are canna-curious, Portugal became the first country in the world in 2001 to legalise the use of all drugs, and started treating drug users as sick people, instead of criminals. The South American nation of Uruguay followed suit in 2013. Now as legal cannabis goes global, more and more nations are coming out of the green closet. Canada's historic decision to end 90 years of prohibition, being the first G7 nation to fully legalize, could soon lead to a domino effect. Canadian medical cannabis companies now export product to countries including Australia, Argentina, South Africa and Germany. Canadian exports also supplement Italy's only legal supply, cultivated by the military.

Israel, a leader in bio and agricultural technology, could emerge as a research hub, but the government has been slow to allow export permits, forcing companies to look elsewhere. According to an unconfirmed report in the Israeli media, Donald Trump called the Israeli prime minister, Benjamin Netanyahu, to object to the industry. Colombia, a nation ravaged by decades of drug-related wars, is now seeking to become a growing centre, while in France two cafes which opened in Paris to sell CBD, were quickly raided and shuttered by police.

Greece and Jamaica have both legalized medical cannabis and are considering cannabis tourism to boost their economies. Jamaica has also legalized it for Sectarians, one on the only recent cannabis law which references religious use. But the country is emerging as a "hemp superpower", with Chinese farmers cashing in on the non-psychoactive cannabis crop, which textile factories buy for its fibre. 100 years ago most of China, from plain to plateau was covered in carefully cultivated opium plants. Most of these have now been replaces by millions of hectares of tobacco plants. In a hundred years from now will the lands that stretch from Hong Kong to the Himalayas be covered in cannabis?

The United Kingdom

Legalisation hit the news in England recently when Charlotte Caldwell returned from Canada with six-month supply of cannabis oil, the most effective medicine she'd found for her young child's epilepsy. She declared the medicine, to British border officials, who immediately confiscated it. This was particularly ironic as the oil in question known as Epidiolex was developed by GW Pharmaceuticals, a British biopharmaceutical company, well-known for its multiple sclerosis treatment Sativex. Unable to take his medicine, Billy was admitted just a few days later to hospital in "life threatening" condition. Sajid Javid, the UK home minister, was forced to issue an emergency license to allow doctors to treat Billy with cannabis oil.

The case sparked an outcry, and Javid called for a review of the UK's medical cannabis policy which recommended that clinicians should be able to prescribe medical cannabis. Inevitably, talk about full legalization has followed and according to recent polls, 82% of Britons support legalizing medical cannabis and 51% support full legalization.

Australia

At the time of writing a proposal to legalise cannabis, and allow people to get high off their own supply is being reviewed by a tripartisan health committee in the National Assembly. There is a little squabbling going one between the different parties as to who is going to be seen as the most progressive, but both Labour and the Greens support the bill to legalise cannabis in principle, which will probably be passed this summer.

New Zealand

The government announced late last year that medical cannabis would be allowed, and the country is due to hold a national referendum by 2020 on whether to legalize and regulate adult use of cannabis. The exact language and scope of the referendum question remain unclear.

Mexico

Ravaged by drug war violence and corruption, Mexico decriminalized the possession of small amounts of cannabis and other drugs in 2009. With the blessing of President Lopez Obrador, a series of Mexico Supreme Court rulings beginning in 2015 began laying the groundwork for cannabis legalization by holding that people should have the right to grow and distribute cannabis for personal use. The new president's party controls both houses of Mexico's Congress, which bodes very well for ease of passage.

The Netherlands

Hoping to keep pot users away from dealers of harder drugs, the Netherlands in the late 1970s began allowing "coffee shops" to sell cannabis. The shops remain a popular attraction, especially in Amsterdam, but the drug remains illegal elsewhere in the country and purveyors have long complained about having to resort to the black market to obtain it since cultivation is outlawed. Critics say the system has allowed criminal organizations and money laundering to persist. That could be changing. The new Dutch government has committed to a trial program by which it will license a producer to provide cannabis in six to 10 cities.

South Africa

South Africa's Supreme Court ruled last month that adults can use cannabis and grow it for personal consumption -- in private.

Italy

Reform advocates have been promoting cannabis legalization in Italy for years, without success. But in late 2016, a law legalizing production of hemp -- a very low-THC version of cannabis favoured for myriad industrial uses -- took effect. Since then, the dried flowers of those plants have been sold in some shops, giving supporters new hope for future legalization efforts.

A cannabis regulation measure has been making its way through Italy's parliament and still needs support from more legislators. Italy could be a "dark horse in the race to be the first country to legalize in Europe," Rolles says.

The United States

With its northern neighbour legalizing and its southern neighbour mulling it, can the world's most influential proponent of the drug war be far behind?

While President Donald Trump has said he would likely

support a congressional effort to ease the federal prohibition, his attorney general, Jeff Sessions, is a cannabis critic and legalization opponent.

The longer the US delays, the longer the country misses out on potentially significant economic opportunities. US cannabis companies and operators who are being snubbed by the US banking system, are already looking to Canada to secure financing. Canadian investment bankers are more than willing to work with cannabis companies looking to grow from one state to another. Companies such as the MGO-ELLO Alliance are promising much-needed A-to-Z services to get finances in order, from audits to taxes and everything in between.

Thailand

At the end of 2018 Thailand became the first country in Asia to legalise medical cannabis. Every South East Asia country has long been in denial about the popularity recreational use of cannabis by tourists. The fact is that cosmopolitan international visitors are often looking for exotic thrills. The Thai government rarely talks about the Thai sex industry except to deny its entire existence but the physical evidence of huge red light entertainment areas in Bangkok, Phuket and Pattaya quickly dispel this myth. Prostitution is prohibited but hardly ever prosecuted, making its existence an open secret. Pimps, hookers and their johns are openly tolerated because of the incomes they bring in from abroad. While turning a blind eye to the sex trade, trafficking and abuse, anybody caught with a harmless bit of ganja is persecuted to the full effect of the law. Worse yet, this leverage is often put to very profitable use by the corrupt local police who run a very nice racket in entrapment. Just as there are no official figures on how many are attracted to Asia by the sex industry, governments refuse to even acknowledge that any one particular demographic is attracted by the local availability of cannabis.

As yet, it is unfortunately unclear how the new laws will actually work in practice. It is widely suspected that the new law is simply a carrot dangled in front of poor uneducated Thai peasants, in the hope that they will support the military junta in the upcoming elections. Whether any real changes will actually be made, remains to be seen.

Recent legalisation laws have prompted a very negative reaction from some countries. Japan has given its residents in Canada a stern warning saying the possession and purchase of the drug is not only illegal in Japan, but "may be applied ... in foreign countries. Of course, the harshest regimes including Saudi and China make it illegal for anybody to have any THC in their systems.

South Korea is the first East Asian country to legalize medical cannabis, but rather than being one of the most liberal approaches to cannabis, it is actually one of the world's most restrictive medical cannabis programs. The authorities will only allow the import of medical cannabis products that have received government approval from major world powers like the U.S. or the U.K and only if no alternative medicine exists in the country. This restriction currently limits imports to two synthetic cannabinoids – Marinol and Cesamet – and two cannabis-derived pharmaceuticals – Sativex and Epidiolex. Patients wishing to use cannabis treatments must submit their medical records, a full diagnosis of their condition, and a doctor's note stating that medical cannabis is the only possible treatment for their ailment.

The head of the narcotics crime investigation division warned that Korea will actively prosecute Korean nationals who partake in Canada with prison sentences up to five years in prison or a fine of up to 50 million won, around $57,000. In response, the Prime Minister of Canada has responded by implementing a jail term for Canadians that consume kimchi, which is apparently a highly dangerous 'gateway cabbage.'

The concept of cannabis being a gateway drug has always been one of the fallacies repeated again and again by the War on Drugs. Even so, it is the nature of human beings to evolve and develop, and so I think that it is therefore inevitable that consumers will demand even more effective chemical stimulants and aphrodisiacs in the future. I personally side with the Shulgins when they state that a drug is pretty much worthless if you cannot either communicate when you are affected by it, or also to make love having taken it. After all these are the two primary characteristics of consciousness that make us human, or at least I think so. Sasha did not like compounds that he describes as being too 'sparkly', and I would agree with that too. What you really want is something that opens up your natural creativity, not something that gets you so high and out of it that you are no longer physically able to operate. So this means that we are looking for the equivalent of the Goldilocks effect. Not something that turns you into a zombie, nor something that has you tripping away like an out-of-control shaman, but something just in between, where you are still able to retain some modicum of self control and self awareness. This is probably why natural substances such as mushrooms and weed are so eternally popular. Ideally these effects should have you thinking about questions like "How is this affecting my mind, and "Where exactly is my mind located?" If an experience has you seeing colours that you cannot recognise and to which you cannot put names, then you are probably somewhere around the ideal level.

2C-B is the archetypal Shulgin psychedelic. It possesses all the qualities he searched for throughout his career. 2C-B is potent, warm, corporeal, associative, shows no signs of physical toxicity, and has a short duration, ideal for psychotherapy. It is also extremely "erotic." Shulgin said, "If there is anything ever found to be an effective aphrodisiac, it will probably be patterned after 2C-B in structure." It was, unfortunately, made illegal after a brief stint as a legal sex enhancer.

Further Reading

Sex Pot: The Marijuana Lover's Guide to Gettin' It On

by Mamakind

This long time writer for Cannabis Culture magazine, Cannabis Health Journal and Skunk Magazine can certainly write and with what an imagination. She speaks very openly about sex and pot and subjects we all think about but probably are not too comfortable with ourselves. The only problem is that it is written very much from an insider's point of view. This is hardly surprising considering that she founded one of the very first medical cannabis dispensaries (the Sunshine Coast Compassion Club Society), but it does sometimes make the content rather inaccessible and difficult to understand for the average non-hippy suburbanite. I certainly enjoyed the personal experiences shared and new learned many new things about kink but felt very much like an outsider, looking into a very niche counter culture.

The Biotechnology of Cannabis Sativa 2nd Edition: Extreme Publications, Inc. (April 20, 2014)

With the therapeutic effects of cannabis becoming realized by industry, some have predicted that in 2016 the market for cannabis-based drugs will be just under $30 billion. Several major companies are seriously working towards developing pharmaceutical products from cannabis, and more companies are realizing the potential and joining the cannabis rush. Undoubtedly, cannabis biotechnology will be crucial to delivering medical and recreational needs for millions of people.

In this edition, some sections become quite technical, allowing the readers to immerse themselves in a deeper level of understanding. Molecular genetics, manipulation of cannabinoid production, tissue culture, transgenic systems, molecular details of gene transfer, cannabis genomics, and bioinformatics are only a few of the emerging sciences that have been included in this edition. Although much of the presentation is in a form that should be pleasantly digestible to almost any reader, there are several sections where technical details were necessarily included.

The target reading group, as it has been argued all books must have one, is therefore quite diverse. Those concerned with how the cannabis landscape is evolving will find this book highly informative. Cannabis growers and consumers will understand why holding on to their seeds might be important. Students of plant biotechnology will find the ideas and techniques useful in guiding their own research questions. At the same time, this is not a textbook and instead delivers the study of plant biotechnology in a flavourful way. Considering the diverse interests of researchers working around the world on cannabis and the excellent, detailed published research articles currently available, much can be said about the biotechnology of cannabis. While legalization is changing who is consuming cannabis, biotechnology is redefining cannabis. Thus, this world-famous plant has the potential to take several new paths that are filled with uncertainty. At least for the moment, the only certainty is that cannabis will never be the same.

Sex at Dawn: The Prehistoric Origins of Modern Sexuality

by Christopher Ryan and Cacilda Jethá

The authors argue that human beings evolved in exceedingly promiscuous pre-agrarian hunter-gatherer societies in which sexual interaction was a shared resource, much like food, child care, and group defence. In opposition to what the authors see as the "standard narrative" of human sexual evolution, they contend that having multiple sexual partners was common and accepted in the environment of evolutionary adaptedness. Sex was relatively promiscuous, and paternity was not a concern, in a similar way to the mating system of bonobos. According to the book, sexual interactions strengthened the bond of trust in the groups; far from causing jealousy, social equilibrium and reciprocal obligation was strengthened by playful sexual interactions.

The first two-thirds of the book focused primarily on history, past studies and how people felt about sex (or sexuality) and mating. The last third pulled all this information together and compared it to how we feel today, in our recent past, and how we may feel about it in the future. Once I finished the book I didn't feel like I was just told what to think, but simply had a lot more to think about.

The book generated a great deal of publicity in the popular press, where it was met with generally positive reviews. The book was praised by syndicated sex-advice columnist Dan Savage, who wrote: "Sex At Dawn is the single most important book about human sexuality since Alfred Kinsey unleashed Sexual Behaviour in the Human Male on the American public in 1948.

Newsweek's Kate Daily wrote, "This book takes a swing at pretty much every big idea on human nature: that poverty is an inevitable consequence of life on earth, that mankind is by nature brutish, and, most important, that humans evolved to be monogamous. ... [Sex at Dawn] sets out to destroy almost each and every notion of the discipline, turning the field on its head and taking down a few big names in science in the process. ... Funny, witty, and light."

Carefully researched and thoughtfully and humorously presented, this book will inspire you to reassess your ideas about humanity's basic urges, and is very different from the Jared Diamond-type theories that are so prevalent today. It was especially eye-opening to learn about the suppression strategies employed by society to desexualize women. It is considered a must read for every sexuality educator, therapist, researcher and anyone else seriously interested in the subject. Say good bye to shame and ignorance and say hello to greater understanding of our sexual needs

A number of scholars from related academic disciplines were critical of the book's methodology, even complaining that the language is not scientific. It is clear that these inhabitants of the ivory towers were suffering from severe sour grapes and spent far too much time reading obscure scientific journals to comprehend that a modern best-seller needs to be enjoyable to read.

Ryan originally tried to publish the book with academic publisher Oxford University Press, but it was rejected for publication after 2 of 3 peer reviews were negative during the publisher's internal peer-review process. It is not hard to understand why "Sex at Dawn" has been embraced by sexologists while the personally threatened primatologists and anthropologists have been noticeably cooler in their reception. The book is like a bomb thrown not only against the very notion of monogamy but also against the standard narrative in anthropology that pair-bonding is universal in human societies because women trade sexual access for food and protection.

Sex at Dusk: Lifting the Shiny Wrapping from Sex at Dawn

by Lynn Saxon

Using predominantly the same sources, Sex at Dusk is a vigorous rebuttal of Sex at Dawn shrouds claiming the Rousseau-ian sexual idylls only existed in the overheated libidinous imaginations of the authors. Saxon sometimes wrongly assumes that Ryan and Jetha are making arguments that they are not actually making. This leads her to sometimes criticize them on areas she actually agrees with them. Dawn is a much more entertaining read, but Dusk is far more rigorous in its arguments - after all, it's arguments are based on the arguments made by all evolutionary biologists. That said, Saxon misrepresents some of their arguments. Dusk makes too many assumptions whenever Dawn fails to make its arguments completely explicit.

As an author myself, it is tempting to think that Saxon simply thought to herself, "Wow, that Sex at Dawn has become an instant best-seller. What can I write on a related theme that will appeal to a similar audience. In a digital world where sales are based largely on Amazon algorithms, this writing strategy is all too common.

Supplement to the Voyages of Bougainville

Denis Diderot

Written way back in 1772, the Supplement spans five chapters in the form of a dialogue between two people, but the characters and setting varies. Chapter two features a Tahitian Elder addressing a Captain Bougainville, while chapters three and four are between a villager named Orou and his European chaplain guest. In each of the dialogues, Diderot aligns one character with European culture and the other with Tahitian culture for the purpose of contrasting the two. By comparing these two societies, Diderot is able to produce moral statements about the way that people live. Denis Diderot believed that universal progress depends largely on a sexual energy that fuels the universe. This concept greatly influenced Diderot's views on human sexuality. His involvement in Enlightenment movements such as sensualism, vitalism and materialism also helped him developed his ideas about human sexuality. Since nature favours procreation, laws and rules should not restrain the sexuality of men and women. Diderot's critique of 18th century French society, especially its rules controlling human sexuality, can especially be seen in the Supplément au Voyage de Bougainville.

Tahitian people are governed by nature and portrayed as happy and content. They also have less restrictions on their sexual conduct because men and women are not obligated to marry before having a child together. People can have sex with the opposite gender in order to procreate, which is nature's intended purpose for humans. In Tahiti, women were not considered property of any man nor shamed for having a child before marriage. French women on the other hand were no longer free to satisfy their own desires after marriage, especially sexual ones, and had to adhere to the commands of their "bourgeois patriarchs."

Straight: The Surprisingly Short History of Heterosexuality

by Hanne Blank

In this fascinating study of how Western views of what it means to be 'straight,' Blank offers numerous intriguing, thought-provoking argument that love and passion are not defined by biology. Instead, she describes how sexuality has changed over the past two centuries and continues to change and offers the provocative solution that soon we will move on from our present fixation on the binary to a more fluid understanding. This is a meticulously researched romp through the history of 'heterosexuality'—that pesky orthodoxy still looming over Western culture like smog, which may in fact be merely "a particular configuration of sex and power in a particular historical moment."

This is a wonderful history that diligently researches a word that many use, but few really understand. A compelling story of how and why we, as Western society (there is little to no mention of other cultures), refer to and think in certain ways about the heterosexual/homosexual dichotomy. What would it mean to dispense with our current categories of sexual identity? As entertaining as it is profoundly enlightening, this book might even cause you to redefine your own sexual orientation.

Sex, Time, and Power: How Women's Sexuality Shaped Human Evolution

by Leonard Shlain

Shlain brings his experience as a surgeon and his life-long interest in evolutionary theory to this question: Why is global society so shot through with misogyny and patriarchy? Everyone wonders, "why am I here"? This book answers that question through the ages - young women, middle-aged women, older women, all have a grand purpose in the design of life.

This is a conversation on the subject of male/female dynamics, where the author pieces together facts, like a puzzle, in order to build a coherent theory of what might have happened. Determinations that shape the relationship between men and women. Schlain approaches the subject of human sexual reproductive systems from his early med school curiosity of why women have a standard 15% less iron count than men. He explores multiple theories when considering why we circumcise men, why women need to couple, why we might have evolved the G-spot orgasm, the value and function of the post menopausal woman/ grandmother in society, etc. why is there "marriage" - one man, one woman. And how did that get passed along as our accepted form of mating, why not one husband and lots of wives? Although dense, this is an easy and enjoyable read. And I never would have dreamed that the woman's monthly cycle has such a huge impact on....so many things! Fascinating stuff.....!

The Ethical Slut: A Guide to Infinite Sexual Possibilities

by Dossie Easton and Catherine A. Liszt

The monogamous married life is not for everyone and this is a great start for anyone interested in polyamory. This is a comprehensive, no-holds-barred guide for anyone who dreams of having all the sex and love and friendship they want. Here are the skills you need for successful - and ethical - sluthood, from scheduling dates to handling jealousy, finding partners to resolving conflict, raising children to caring for your health. If you've ever envisioned a universe beyond traditional lifetime monogamy, this is the book for you. Definitely a hedonistic focus that places value on personal satisfaction regardless of societal mores. This book is a great resource for people new to this lifestyle, being safe but also being free to live a life true to yourself and your own wishes/values, not those placed on you by others.

When it comes to audio recommendations, generally speaking, it is probably better for each of us to choose our own personal soundtrack to accompany our own sexual adventures. We all have very different tastes when it comes to a sensual bedroom soundtrack, ranging from Idris Mohammed and Fela Kuti, all the way to Nick Drake and Miles Davies.

One recording that I do want to mention specifically here though, is Louise Huebner's 'Seduction Through Witchcraft' released on Warner Brothers Records in 1969. With a psychedelic backing track by the electronic music pioneer Louis Barron (who created the original Forbidden Planet soundtrack way back in 1956, which still sounds suitably extraterrestrial, even today) the 'Official Witch of Los Angeles' dramatically narrated a selection of love and sex spells accented with mystical sound effects and an echoing, seductive vocal style.

This reverb-heavy collection of erotic incantations centred around "charms of seduction and sexual power", and is a mesmerizing and entertaining listen from start to finish. Best listened to by candlelight, obviously.

Huebner adapted much of her best-selling book of the same name for this auditory Book of Shadows, which portrayed witches as capricious and orgiastic individuals.

111

"Enchanters need orgies. The orgies will help you generate the electrical and magnetic impulses you will need to cast spells."

The album later gained an even wider audience when excerpts were spliced into a 1973 David Bowie bootleg. The spacey, synthy, mystery music, and a dark, seductive voice intoning the correct conditions under which to stage an orgy seemed to blend perfectly with Bowie's Ziggy-era message.

This sixth generation sorceress spoke a litany of different languages including Latin, French, and Italian, and was often invited to assist in crime detection. On July 21, 1968, she was to demonstrate her craft at the opening ceremony of Twelve Summer Sunday Concerts in the Hollywood Bowl. The enchantment was meant to increase the sexual vitality of the entire County, including 11.000 people who were present at the event. Huebner, dressed in a long silver robe, passed out red candles, chalk, salt and garlic, and led a mass ritual to cast a spell over Los Angeles County, in order to raise its "romantic and emotional vitality." The spell consisted of a group incantation: "Light the flame/Bright the fire/red is the colour of desire." which was led by Louise Huebner on stage.

As to whether the spell worked, well, it might only be a coincidence, but the San Fernando Valley which is now a large urban district of Los Angeles County went on to be a pioneering region for producing adult films in the 1970s. It grew to become home of the multi billion-dollar pornography industry and was soon known as the porn capital of the world. At its height, nearly 90 percent of all legally distributed pornographic films made in the United States were either filmed in or produced by studios based in the San Fernando Valley.

Of course, not all of your weed-related experience needs to be sexual. Music is enhanced beyond all recognition by cannabis, and in this day and age, when you can store an entire archive of artists and genres onto a cheap smart phone, a few hours inside a pair of headphones can become a truly mystical experience. If you have never had the experience of a piece of music bringing you to gushing tears, then this is something that you really must try.

More Titles From the Borderland Press

Darby Jones

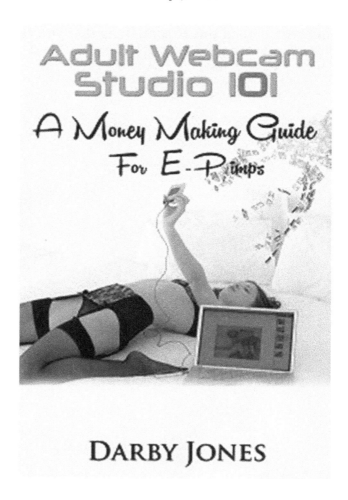

Adult Webcam Studio 101 - A Money Making Guide for ePimps

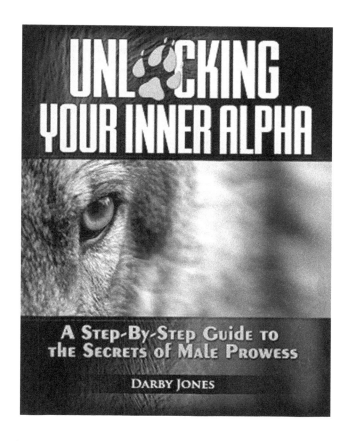

Unlocking Your Inner Alpha - A Step-by-Step Guide to the Secrets of Male Prowess

FORTHCOMING

Bianca Latimer

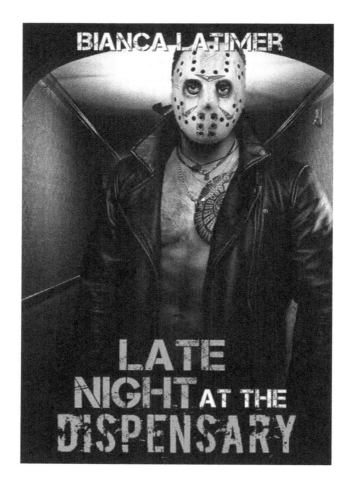

Late Night at the Dispensary

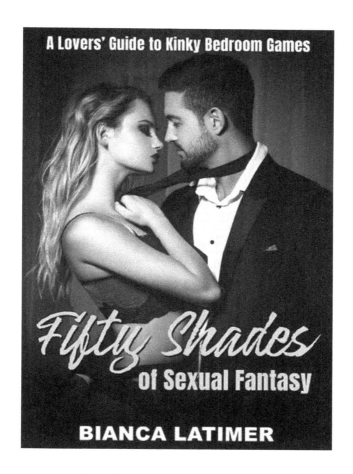

Fifty Shades of Sexual Fantasy

Palmer Eldritch

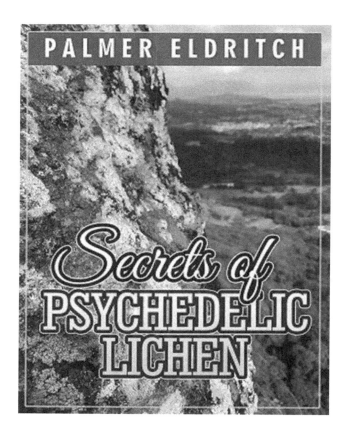

Secrets of Psychoactive Lichen

Darby Jones

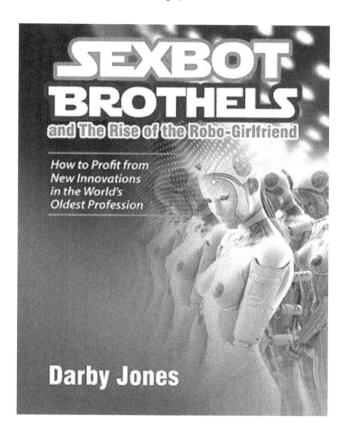

Sexbot Brothels and the Rise of the Robo-Girlfriend

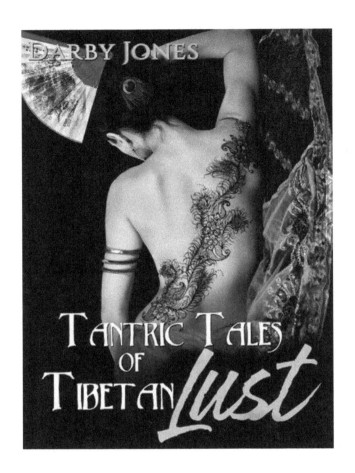

Tantric Tales of Tibetan Lust

About the Author

Bianca has always enjoyed in-depth research work, and her non-fiction work shows that she is both inventive and resourceful.

It was not until recently that Bianca discovered that she had a hidden talent for hot and steamy erotica, with wildly over-the-top scenarios and wickedly taboo relationships. Having worked in the same, quiet library since she left school, nobody would dream from looking at her, that her imagination is bursting with sinfully hot tales of love, lust and forbidden passions. Behind those gold rimmed spectacles, there lie untold universes of aggressive alphas and unapologetic bad boys.

Unfortunately, she is is far less skilled when it comes to dealing with the opposite sex in real life. In fact, she is far better with animals than she is with people. When she is not writing or working, she can usually be found down at the local dog pound, helping to take care of the city's unwanted strays.

If you would like to chat, discuss or even hang out, Bianca can be contacted at biancalatimer2020@gmail.com. She loves hearing from readers and always replies to any email received.

Printed in the USA
CPSIA information can be obtained
at www.ICGtesting.com
LVHW050929050923
757197LV00032B/359